AF553277

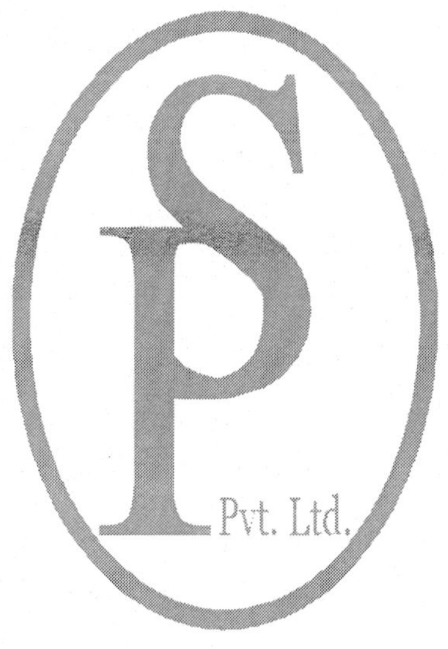

Handbook of Practical Human Anatomy And Physiology

Vishal S. Gulecha

Manoj S. Mahajan

Chandrashekhar D. Upasani

2019

Studium Press (India) Pvt. Ltd.

Handbook of Practical Human Anatomy And Physiology

ISBN: 978-93-85046-59-9

Published by:

Studium Press (India) Pvt. Ltd.
4735/22, 2nd Floor, Prakash Deep Building
(Near Delhi Medical Association),
Ansari Road, Darya Ganj, New Delhi-110 002
Tel.: + 91-11-43240200-15 (15 lines); Fax: 91-11-43240215
E-mail: pubdir@studiumpress.in

Printed at India

Foreword

This book *Handbook of Practical Human Anatomy and Physiology* provides valuable information and covers the necessary components to learn anatomy and physiology practically.

I hope the present book will enable the students to grasp the essential features of practical Anatomy and Physiology and to achieve an understanding in relation to complex concepts of the course.

It is my expectation that this book will provide an effective learning experience and a resource for all the learners especially to the students and other users.

On behalf of all authors, I welcome suggestions, criticism from the readers, Professionals and students.

Dr. Chandrashekhar D. Upasani

About Author(s)

Dr. Vishal S. Gulecha

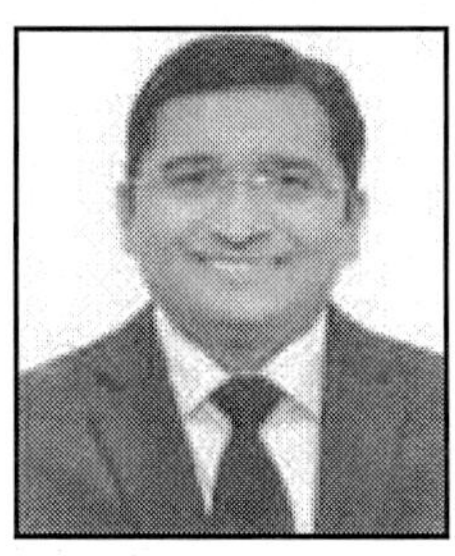

Dr. Vishal S. Gulecha is working as an Assistant Professor, Department of Pharmacology at SNJB's Shriman Sureshdada Jain College of Pharmacy, Chandwad (M. S.). He has persued B. Pharm (2005) and Masters Degree in Pharmacology in 2007 from the Pune University. He has completed his Ph.D. from Dr. MGR Medical University, Chennai (2012). He has 12 years of teaching experience. He has published several research articles and reviews in the national and international journal of repute. He is recipient of different awards for presentation of research work at various conferences and symposia. Also he has received grants for research from Savitribai Phule Pune University.

Mr. Manoj S. Mahajan

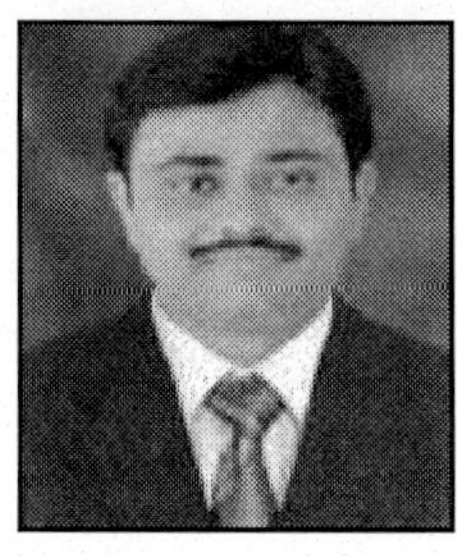

Mr. Manoj S. Mahajan is working as an Assistant Professor, Department of Pharmacology at SNJB's Shriman Sureshdada Jain College of Pharmacy, Chandwad (M. S.). He has persued B. Pharm (2006) and M. Pharm in Pharmacology (2008) from the Pune University. He has 11 years of teaching experience. He has published several research articles and reviews in the national and international journals and presented research work at various national and international conferences. He has received grants for research from Savitribai Phule Pune University. He is currently perusing his Ph D. from Savitribai Phule Pune University.

Dr. Chandrashekhar D. Upasani

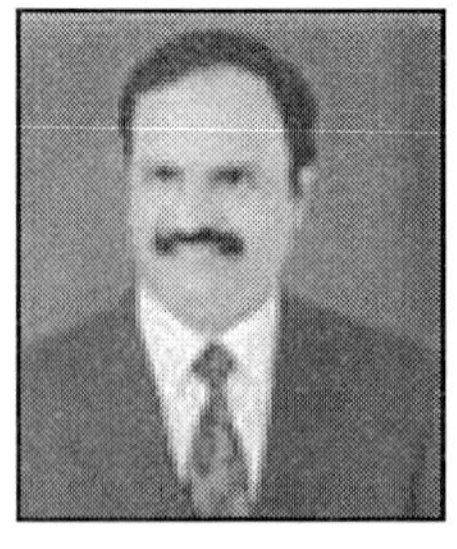

Dr. Chandrashekhar D. Upasani is Professor and Principal at the SNJB's Shriman Sureshdada Jain College of Pharmacy, Chandwad (M. S.). He had more than 22 years of teaching and administrative experience. He is former Dean and BOS Chairman of faculty of Pharmacy, Savitribai Phule Pune University, Pune. He is also associated with other Universities of repute as BOS member and on other administrative bodies. He is approved Ph.D. guide of SPPU, Pune. More than 15 students awarded Ph.D. under his guideship. He has organized several National and International Conferences and Seminars. He has delivered several invited talk in various Conferences. He has completed major research projects and published more than 5 books.

The authors of this book are recipient of prestigious NN Dutta Award given for the research papers published in *Indian Journal of Pharmacology* by Indian National. The condition for this award is the work must have been carried out in an Indian Laboratory. The prize was given to the paper entitled, "Screening of *Ficus religiosa* leaves fractions for analgesic and anti-inflammatory activities" published in Ind. J. Pharmacol, 2011; 43:662-666, in scientific session at IPSCON-2012-XXXXV Annual Conference of Indian Pharmacological Society & International Conference on Navigating Pharmacology towards safe and Effective therapy held at Nagpur on 5th to 7th January 2013.

Preface

The content of this book *Handbook of Practical Human Anatomy and Physiology* are designed and conforms to the syllabi of Human Anatomy & Physiology laid down by the Pharmacy Council of India, which is mandatory and is followed by all Pharmacy institutes.

This book is intended for Pharmacy and Medical students but will be useful to others who need concise knowledge of the subject like Medical laboratory technicians, Nurses and paramedical scientists.

The book consists of different sections and related experiments which will give in depth knowledge of the subject to the beginners.

It includes experiments on basics of Anatomy and Physiology to learn about human body, anatomical terms, directional terms and other relevant concepts in a simple way using figures.

The book also focuses on histology, the study of four basic types of tissues and their subtypes including microscopic features of the each type tissues along with their locations and function with diagrammatic representations.

The users of this book will find the experiments on human skeleton and its divisions, structure of bone and different bones associated with the divisions of skeleton.

It is also inclusive of study of different systems of human body with anatomical and histological features of different associated organs.

The ultimate goal of this book is to help the students to understand the principle, correct use of apparatus with proper technique while performing various experiments especially those related to hematology.

We have tried our best to give better to our students through lucid, clear and fine language throughout the text. Questions and answers section is provided with most of the experiments for easy learning and to initiate a logical thinking. It is also helpful for the learners to face viva during examinations.

May this book act as the medium for the students to gain and grasp the essence of the concepts in practical anatomy and physiology, and ease their journey of learning this complex but extremely interesting science.

Table of Contents

Experiment No. 1

Aim: To Study Body as a Whole

***Key words*:** Definitions, Level of Structural Organization, Body Cavities, Membranes, Directional Terms, Body Planes and Sections

DEFINITIONS

Anatomy

The word anatomy is derived from a Greek word "*Anatome*" meaning to cut up. It is the study of structures that make up the body and how those structures relate with each other. The study of anatomy includes many sub specialties. These are Gross anatomy, Microscopic anatomy, Developmental anatomy and Embryology.

***Gross anatomy*:** Studies body structure without microscope.

***Systemic anatomy*:** Studies functional relationships of organs within a system

***Regional anatomy*:** Studies body part regionally.

Both systemic and regional approaches may be used to study gross anatomy.

***Microscopic anatomy (Histology)*:** Requires the use of microscope to study tissues that form the various organs of the body.

***Physiology*:** The word physiology derived from a Greek word for study of nature. It is the study of how the body and its part work or function.

Homeostasis

When structure and function are coordinated the body achieves a relative stability of its internal environment called *homeostasis* / staying the same. Although the external environmental changes constantly, the internal environment of a healthy body remains the same within normal limits.

Under normal conditions, homeostasis is maintained by adaptive mechanisms ranging from control center in the brain to chemical substances called hormones that are secreted by various organs directly into the blood streams. Some of the functions controlled by homeostasis mechanisms are blood pressure, body temperature, breathing and heart rate.

Level of structural organization of the body

The human body has different structural levels of organization, starting with atoms molecules and compounds and increasing in size and complexity to cells, tissues, organs and the systems that make up the complete organism.

Chemical level

Atoms molecules and compounds at its simplest level, the body is composed of atoms. The most common elements in living organism are carbon, hydrogen, oxygen, nitrogen phosphorus and sulfur.

Atoms → Molecule → Compounds

Cellular level

The chemicals that make up the body may be divided into two major categories: inorganic and organic.

Inorganic chemicals are usually simple molecules made of one or two elements other than carbon (with a few exceptions). Examples of inorganic chemicals are water (H_2O); oxygen (O_2); one of the exceptions, carbon dioxide (CO_2); and minerals such as iron (Fe), calcium (Ca), and sodium (Na).

Organic chemicals are often very complex and always contain the elements carbon and hydrogen. In this category of organic chemicals are carbohydrates, fats, proteins, and nucleic acids.

The smallest independent units of life. All life depends on the many chemical activities of cells. Some of the basic functions of cell are: growth, metabolism, irritability and reproduction. They are too small to be seen with the naked eye, but when magnified using a microscope different types can be distinguished by their size, shape and the dyes they absorb when stained in the laboratory. Each cell type has become *specialised,* and carries out a particular function that contributes to body needs.

Tissue level: tissue is made up of many similar cells that perform a specific function. The various tissues of the body are divided in to four groups. These are epithelial, connective, nervous and muscle tissue.

***Epithelial tissue*:** Found in the outer layer of skin, lining of organs, blood and lymph vessels and body cavities.

***Connective tissue*:** Connects and supports most part of the body. They constitute most part of skin, bone and tendons.

***Muscle tissue*:** Produces movement through its ability to contract. This constitutes skeletal, smooth and cardiac muscles.

***Nerve tissue*:** Found in the brain, spinal cord and nerves. It responds to various types of stimuli and transmits nerve impulses.

***Organ level*:** Is an integrated collection of two or more kinds of tissue that works together to perform specific function. An organ level is a group of organs that all contribute to a particular function. Examples are the urinary system, digestive system, and respiratory system. In the urinary system, this consists of the kidneys, ureters, urinary bladder, and urethra. These organs all contribute to the formation and elimination of urine.

System level: Is a group of organs that work together to perform major function.

Some organs are part of two organ systems; the pancreas, for example, is both a digestive and an endocrine organ, and the diaphragm is part of both the muscular and respiratory systems. All of the organ systems make up an individual person.

Organism level: The various organs of the body form the entire organism. (Table 1.1)

CAVITIES OF THE BODY

The organs that make up the systems of the body are contained in four *cavities:*

- Cranial
- Thoracic
- Abdominal
- Pelvic

Cranial cavity

The cranial cavity contains the *brain,* and its boundaries are formed by the bones of the skull (cranial bones).

Anteriorly — 1 frontal bone

Laterally — 2 temporal bones

Posteriorly — 1 occipital bone

Superiorly — 1 parietal bones

Inferiorly — 1 sphenoid and 1 ethmoid bone and parts of the frontal, temporal and occipital bones.

Table 1.1: System of human body

System	*Organs*	*Functions*
Integumentary	Skin, subcutaneous tissue	Is a barrier to pathogens and chemicals Prevents excessive water loss
Skeletal	Bones, ligaments	Supports the body Protects internal organs and red bone marrow Provides a framework to be moved by muscles
Muscular	Muscles, tendons	Moves the skeleton Produces heat
Nervous	Brain, nerves, eyes, ears	Interprets sensory information Regulates body functions such as movement by means of electrochemical impulses
Endocrine	Thyroid gland, pituitarygland, pancreas	Regulates body functions such as growth and reproduction by means of hormones Regulates day-to-day metabolism by means of hormones
Circulatory	Heart, blood, arteries	Transports oxygen and nutrients to tissues and removes waste products
Lymphatic	Spleen, lymph nodes	Returns tissue fluid to the blood • Destroys pathogens that enter the body and provides immunity
Respiratory	Lungs, trachea, larynx, diaphragm	Exchanges oxygen and carbon dioxide between the air and blood
Digestive	Stomach, colon, liver, pancreas	Changes food to simple chemicals that can be absorbed and used by the body
Urinary	Kidneys, urinary bladder, urethra	Removes waste products from the blood Regulates volume and pH of blood and tissue fluid
Reproductive	*Female*: ovaries, uterus *Male*: testes, prostate gland	Produces eggs or sperm *In women*, provides a site for the developing embryo-fetus

Thoracic cavity

This cavity is situated in the upper part of the trunk. Its boundaries are formed by a bony framework and supporting muscles

Anteriorly — The sternum and costal cartilages of the ribs

Laterally — 12 pairs of ribs and the intercostal muscles

Posteriorly — The thoracic vertebrae and the intervertebral discs between the bodies of the vertebrae

Superiorly — The structures forming the root of the neck

Inferiorly — The diaphragm, a dome-shaped muscle

Contents

The main organs and structures contained in the thoracic cavity are

- The trachea, 2 bronchi, 2 lungs
- The heart, aorta, superior and inferior vena cava, numerous other blood vessels
- The oesophagus
- Lymph vessels and lymph nodes
- Nerves.

The *mediastinum* is the name given to the space between the lungs including the structures found there, such as the heart, oesophagus and blood vessels.

Abdominal cavity

This is the largest cavity in the body and is oval in shape. It is situated in the main part of the trunk and its boundaries are:

Superiorly — Tthe diaphragm, which separates it from the thoracic cavity

Anteriorly — The muscles forming the anterior abdominal wall

Posteriorly —*The* lumbar vertebrae and muscles forming the posterior abdominal wall

Laterally — The lower ribs and parts of the muscles of the abdominal wall

Inferiorly — The pelvic cavity with which it is continuous.

Contents

Most of the space in the abdominal cavity is occupied by the organs and glands involved in the digestion and absorption of food. These are:

- The stomach, small intestine and most of the large intestine
- The liver, gall bladder, bile ducts and pancreas.

  Other structures include:
- The spleen
- 2 kidneys and the upper part of the ureters
- 2 adrenal (suprarenal) glands
- Numerous blood vessels, lymph vessels, nerves
- Lymph nodes.

Pelvic cavity

The pelvic cavity is roughly funnel shaped and extends from the lower end of the abdominal cavity. The boundaries are:

Superiorly — It is continuous with the abdominal cavity

Anteriorly — The pubic bones

Posteriorly — The sacrum and coccyx

Laterally — The innominate bones

Inferiorly — The muscles of the pelvic floor.

Contents

The pelvic cavity contains the following structures:

- Sigmoid colon, rectum and anus
- Some loops of the small intestine
- Urinary bladder, lower parts of the ureters and the urethra
- In the female, the organs of the reproductive system: the uterus, uterine tubes, ovaries and vagina
- In the male, some of the organs of the reproductive system: the prostate gland, seminal vesicles, spermatic cords, deferent ducts (vas deferens), ejaculatory ducts and the urethra (common to the reproductive and urinary systems).

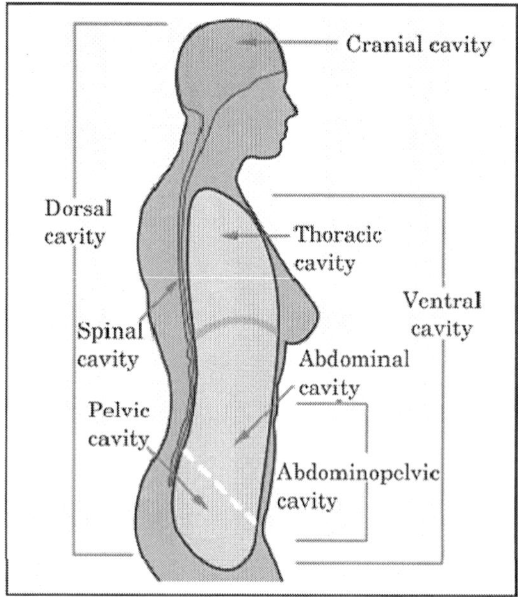

Fig. 1.1: Cavities of body

MEMBRANES

Membranes are sheets of tissue that cover or line surfaces or that separate organs or parts (lobes) of organs from one another. Many membranes produce secretions that have specific functions. The two major categories of membranes are epithelial membranes and connective tissue membranes.

EPITHELIAL MEMBRANES

There are two types of epithelial membranes, serous and mucous. Each type is found in specific locations within the body and secretes a fluid. These fluids are called serous fluid and mucus. (Fig. 1.2: Epithelial membrane).

Serous Membranes

Serous membranes are sheets of simple squamous epithelium that line some closed body cavities and cover the organs in these cavities. The *pleural membranes* are the serous membranes of the thoracic cavity. The parietal pleura lines the chest wall and the

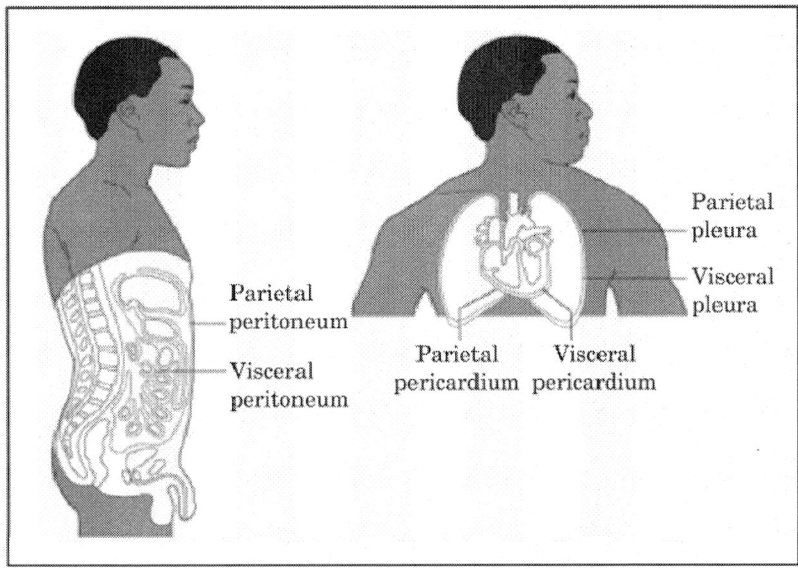

Fig. 1.2: Epithelial membrane

visceral pleura covers the lungs. The pleural membranes secrete *serous fluid*, which prevents friction between them as the lungs expand and recoil during breathing. The heart, in the thoracic cavity between the lungs, has its own set of serous membranes. The parietal *pericardium* lines the fibrous pericardium (a connective tissue membrane), and the visceral pericardium, or *epicardium*, is on the surface of the heart muscle. Serous fluid is produced to prevent friction as the heart beats. In the abdominal cavity, the *peritoneum* is the serous membrane that lines the cavity. The *mesentery,* or visceral peritoneum, is folded over and covers the abdominal organs. Here, the serous fluid prevents friction as the stomach and intestines contract and slide against other organs.

Mucous Membranes

Mucous membranes line the body tracts (systems) that have openings to the environment. These are the respiratory, digestive, urinary, and reproductive tracts. The epithelium of a mucous membrane (mucosa) varies with the different organs involved. The mucosa of the esophagus and of the vagina is stratified squamous epithelium; the mucosa of the trachea is ciliated epithelium; the mucosa of the stomach is columnar epithelium.

Synovial Membrane

Unlike to other membranes this membrane does not contain epithelium. Therefore, it is not epithelial membrane. It lines the cavities of the freely movable joints. Like serious membrane it lines structures that do not open to the exterior. Synovial membranes secret synovial fluid that lubricate articular cartilage at the ends of bones as they move at joints. (Fig. 1.3: Synovial membrane)

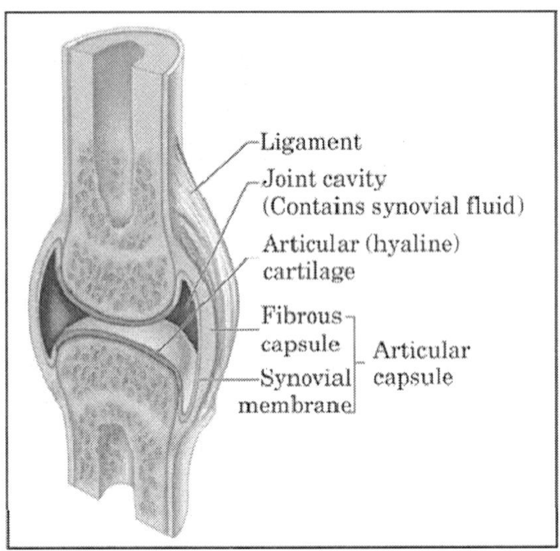

Fig. 1.3: Synovial membrane

Anatomical Terms

The language of anatomy and physiology is very specific. To prevent the confusion, scientists and health-care professionals refer to one standard anatomical position and use a special vocabulary for relating body parts to one another. In the study of anatomy, descriptions of any part of the human body assume that the body is in a specific stance called the *anatomical position*. In the anatomical position, the subject stands erect facing the observer, with the head level and the eyes facing forward. The feet are flat

Table 1.2: Body regions

Body Region	*Description*
Head	Bony portion of head; encloses and protects the brain and gives shape to the face
Skull	
Face	Anterior portion of head not normally covered by scalp
Neck	Body area between head and trunk
Trunk	Central body area to which head and limbs are attached
Chest	Area of trunk between neck and abdomen; contains heart and lungs; diaphragm forms boundary between chest and abdomen
Pelvis	Area of trunk below abdomen; contains internal reproductive
Back	organs and urinary bladder Posterior portion of trunk between neck and buttocks
Upper limb	Curved area where upper limb attaches to upper border of trunk
Shoulder	
Armpit	Under-arm area where upper limb attaches to trunk
Arm	Area of upper limb between shoulder and elbow
Forearm	Area of upper limb between elbow and wrist
Wrist	Portion of hand that connects hand to forearm
Hand	Includes wrist and fingers
Lower limb	Rounded area on posterior surface where thigh attaches to trunk
Buttocks	
Groin	Area on anterior surface marked by a crease where lower limb attaches to the pelvis
Thigh	Area of lower limb above the knee
Leg	Area of lower limb between knee and ankle
Ankle	Portion of foot that connects foot to leg
Foot	Includes ankle and toes

on the floor and directed forward, and the arms are at the sides with the palms turned forward. In the anatomical position, the body is upright. Two terms describe a reclining body. If the body is lying face down, it is in the *prone* position. If the body is lying face up, it is in the *supine* position.

DIRECTIONAL TERMS

To locate various body structures, anatomists use specific *directional terms*, words that describe the position of one body part relative to another. Several directional terms can be grouped in pairs that have opposite meanings. (Table1.3: Directional terms; Fig. 1.4: Directional terms).

Table1.3: Directional terms

Term	*Definition*	*Example of use*
Superior (cranial)	Toward the head	The leg is supper to the foot.
Inferior (caudal)	Toward the feet	The foot is inferior to the leg.
Anterior (ventral)	Toward the front part of the the body	The nose is anterior to the ears.
Posterior (dorsal)	Towards the back of the body	The ears are posterior to the nose.
Medial	Towards the midline of the body	The nose is medial to the eyes.
Lateral	Away from the midline of the body	The eyes are lateral to the nose.
Proximal	Toward (nearer) the trunk of the body or the attached end of a limb.	The shoulder is proximal to the wrist.
Distal	Away (farther) from the trunk of the body or the attached end of a limb.	The wrist is distal to the fore-arm.
Superficial	Nearer the surface of the body	The ribs are superficial to the heart
Deep	Farther from the surface of the body.	The heart is deeper to the ribs.
Peripheral	Away from the central axis of the body.	Peripheral nerves radiate away from the brain and spinal cord
Ipsilateral	On the same side of the body or structure	
Contralateral	On the opposite side of the body or structure	

Body Planes and Sections

Planes are flat surfaces that divide the body or organs in order to expose internal structures. The exposed surfaces produced by planes are called *sections. Sagittal* (*sagitta* = arrow) *planes* pass vertically through the body or organs and divide them into right and left sections *(sagittal sections).* If a plane passes vertically through the midline and divides the body into equal right and left halves, the plane is a *midsagittal plane,* but if a plane divides the body into unequal right and left portions, it is *a parasagittal plane*. *A frontal or coronal plane* passes vertically through the body or organs and produces anterior and posterior sections (*frontal sections*). *A transverse plane* passes horizontally through the body

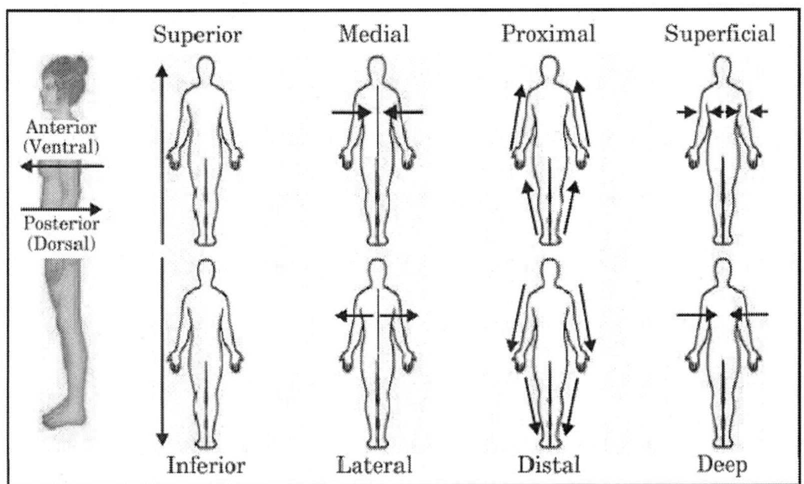

Fig. 1.4: Directional terms

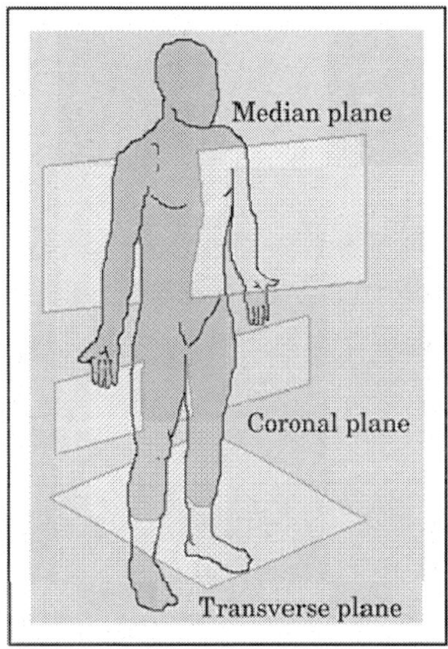

Fig. 1.5: Body planes and sections

and produces superior and inferior sections (*transverse sections or cross-sections*). (Fig. 1.5: *Body Planes and Sections*) *Oblique planes* pass through the body at an angle forming oblique sections. We often look at sections of individual organs, such as blood vessels, intestines, or long bones. Sections that are produced by a plane running along the long axis of a long narrow structure are called *longitudinal sections*. Sections that are produced by a plane running perpendicular to the long axis are called *cross-sections*. Because blood vessels and intestines twist and bend, one body plane may produce longitudinal sections, cross-sections, and oblique sections of these structures.

Experiment No. 2

Aim: To Study the Compound Microscope: Handling, Use & Care

***Key words*:** Parts of Compound Microscope, Methods and use, Routine care and Maintenance

INTRODUCTION

Objects which are smaller than 0.1 mm ordinarily not visible by naked eyes. Therefore, to observe such objects, compound microscope is very helpful. A microscope may be defined as an optical instrument consisting of a lens or combination of lenses for making enlarged or magnified images of minute objects. Magnifying lens is also a type of microscope but its magnifying capacity is very low. Dissecting microscope is also used to visualize tiny things, but it has only one lens. Compound microscope is generally used in the laboratories. A compound light microscope is used to observe small structures such as cells and tissues. The term *compound* refers to the two types of lenses (ocular and objective) that are used simultaneously to magnify the image. The term *light* refers to the necessity of using a light source to view the object. Most human cells must be magnified to be seen by the unaided human eye. The compound light microscope can magnify images up to approximately 1,000 times, depending on the magnifying power of the lenses. Microscopic examination of cells and tissues allows students to observe how cell and tissue structure determines function. Changes in normal cell and tissue structure cause changes in organ function that lead to a disorder or disease. Tissue biopsies are performed to observe whether normal cellular structure has changed, which would indicate the absence or presence of a disorder or disease.

PARTS OF THE COMPOUND MICROSCOPE

There are two commonly used compound microscope- monocular and binocular. Basically, they are the same except that the monocular microscope has one eyepiece (ocular) whereas the binocular microscope has two eyepieces. The parts of the compound microscope can be divided into following four main systems:

1. The support system (the framework)
2. The illumination system
3. The magnification system
4. The adjustment system

THE SUPPORT SYSTEM

The support system is the framework of the microscope that holds its components. The framework consists of following units.

Base: The wide bottom part that supports the microscope. This is horse –shoe shaped(U-shaped) lower portion of the microscope on which the other parts of the microscope lie.

Pillars: Above the U-shaped portion, there is a perpendicular portion known as the pillar

Two upright pillars project upwards from the base, and the handle of the microscope is hinged to the pillars.

Inclination Joint

It is a movable joint, through which the body of the microscope is held to the base by the pillars. The body can be bent at this joint into any inclined position, as desired by the observer, for easier observation. In new models, the body is permanently fixed to the base in an inclined position, thus needing no pillar or joint.

Handle (Arm): It supports the body tube and base of the microscope. This portion is used to hold or carry the microscope. On the base of this, stage is fixed. On the top of the arm body tube of the microscope is fixed and two knobs are fitted. One is for the coarse adjustment and the other for the fine adjustment. These are used for focusing the body tube.

***Body Tube*:** It is usually a vertical tube holding the eyepiece at the top and the revolving nosepiece with the objectives at the bottom. The length of the draw tube is called 'mechanical tube length' and is usually 140-180 mm (mostly 160 mm).

Stage

It is a horizontal platform projecting from the curved arm. It has a hole at the center, upon which the object to be viewed is placed on a slide. Light from the light source below the stage passes through the object into the objective.

Mechanical Stage (Slide Mover)

Mechanical stage consists of two knobs with rack and pinion mechanism. The slide containing the object is clipped to it and moved on the stage in two dimensions by rotating the knobs, so as to focus the required portion of the object.

Revolving Nose-piece

It is a rotatable disc at the bottom of the body tube with three or four objectives screwed to it. The objectives have different magnifying powers. Based on the required magnification, the nose-piece is rotated, so that only the objective specified for the required magnification remains in line with the light path.

THE ILLUMINATION SYSTEM

A microscope cannot function optically without proper illumination. The illumination system provides uniform and soft-bright illumination of the entire field viewed under the microscope. There are six types of illumination system based on which the microscope works: includes Bright-field or light microscope, Dark-field microscope, Fluorescent microscope, Polarizing microscope, Phase-contrast microscope and Interference-contrast microscope.

The illumination system of compound microscope consists of a light source, condenser, and iris diaphragm.

Light Source

The illumination system begins with source of light. Modern microscopes have in-built electric light source in the base. The source is connected to the mains through a regulator, which controls the brightness of the field. But in old models, a mirror is used as the light source. It is fixed to the base by a binnacle, through which it can be rotated, so as to converge light on the object. The mirror is plane on one side and concave on the other.

Internal source

In most modern compound microscope there is a build in light source with an electric lamp, which provides better control of illumination. The lamp housing has a frosted tungsten lamp, which is placed directly under the stage.

External source

In the student compound microscope there in not a build in light source. These microscope use an external source of light. This can be from an electric lamp housed in a lamp box with a window or from the sun. The rays of light are reflected by a mirror towards the object. The mirror is located at the base. The plane mirror is used for the oil-immersion objective whereas the concave mirror is used for the low- and high power objective.

Condenser

The condenser brings the rays of light to a common focus on the object to be examined. It is situated between the mirror and the stage. The condenser can be raised (maximum illumination) and lowered (minimum illumination). It must be centred and adjusted correctly. It has a series of lenses to converge on the object, light rays coming from the light source. After passing through the object, the light rays enter into the objective. The 'light condensing', 'light converging' or 'light gathering' capacity of a condenser is called 'numerical aperture of the condenser'. Similarly, the 'light gathering' capacity of an objective is called 'numerical aperture of the objective'. If the condenser converges light in a wide angle, its numerical aperture is greater and *vice versa*.

If the condenser has such numerical aperture that it sends light through the object with an angle sufficiently large to fill the aperture back lens of the objective, the objective shows its highest numerical aperture. Most common condensers have numerical aperture 1.25.

If the numerical aperture of the condenser is smaller than that of the objective, the peripheral portion of the back lens of the objective is not illuminated and the image has poor visibility. On the other hand, if the numerical aperture of condenser is greater than that of the objective, the back lens may receive too much light resulting in a decrease in contrast.

***There are three types of condensers as follows*:**

(a) Abbe condenser (Numerical aperture=1.25): It is extensively used.

(b) Variable focus condenser (Numerical aperture = 1.25)

(c) Achromatic condenser (Numerical aperture = 1.40): It has been corrected for both spherical and chromatic aberration and is used in research microscopes and photomicrographs.

Iris diaphragm

If light coming from the light source is brilliant and all the light is allowed to pass to the object through the condenser, the object gets brilliantly illuminated and cannot be visualized properly. Therefore, an iris diaphragm is fixed below the condenser to control the amount of light entering into the condenser. It is the iris diaphragm, which is inside the condenser, used to reduce or increase the angle and therefore also the amount of light that passes into the condenser.

THE MAGNIFICATION SYSTEM

The magnification system plays an extremely important role in use of a microscope because it magnifies the image of the object under view. The compound microscope consists of two magnifying lenses, the eyepiece, and the objective. The total magnification obtained in a compound microscope is the product of objective magnification and ocular magnification. The eyepiece forms a magnified image formed by the objective.

Eyepiece

The eyepiece is a drum, which fits loosely into the draw tube. It magnifies the magnified real image formed by the objective to a still greatly magnified virtual image to be seen by the eye.

Usually, each microscope is provided with two types of eyepieces with different magnifying powers (X10 and X25). Depending upon the required magnification, one of the two eyepieces is inserted into the draw tube before viewing. Three varieties of eyepieces are usually available.

Removable eyepieces used to observe the microscope slide. Microscopes with one ocular lens are called *monocular* (*mono-* _ one; *ocu-* _ eye), and those with two ocular lenses are called *binocular* (*bi-* _two). Typically, these lenses magnify an object tenfold (10X). Look at an ocular lens and record the magnification power. One of the ocular lenses may have a *pointer* used to identify a specific area on the slide. A *micrometer*, used to measure the field of view and object size, may also be present in one ocular lens. State whether your microscope has a pointer and/or a micrometer. If it has a pointer or micrometer, give the ocular lens (right or left) in which each is found.

Objective

It is the most important lens in a microscope. Usually three objectives with different magnifying powers are screwed to the revolving nosepiece. The three objectives are:

(a) Low power objective (X 10)

It produces ten times magnification of the object. This objective is used for initial focusing and observations. While using this objective the condenser should be fully lowered and iris diaphragm must be opened slightly. Concave mirror is used to focus the light rays.

(b) High dry objective (X 40 or 45)

It gives a magnification of forty times. This objective is used for more detailed study, as the total magnification. It is used for a broad view of blood films or histological sections prior to their examinations under the oil- immersion objective. This objective is used for broad view of blood films or histologic sections. While using this objective the condenser should be slightly raised and iris diaphragm must be opened partially. Concave mirror is used to focus the light rays.

(c) Oil-immersion objective (X100)

It gives a magnification of hundred times, when immersion oil fills the space between the object and the objective. The objective lens almost rests on the slide. It requires a special type of oil called as immersion oil. The commonly used immersion oil is cedar wood oil which increases the numerical aperture and thus the resolving power of the objective. Light travels through the air at greater speed than the glass and it passes trough the immersion oil at the same speed as through glass. Therefore the oil is used to decrease the speed at which light travels to increase the effective numerical aperture and to decrease the diffraction of light rays. While using this objective the condenser should be fully raised and iris diaphragm must be opened completely. Plane mirror is used to focus the light rays.

A proper illumination of the specimen slide is very essential. However, the students often forget about its importance. The broad rule about illumination (Table 2.1: The broad rule about illumination) is as follows:

Table 2.1: The broad rule about illumination

Objective	*Condenser Position*	*Iris Diaphragm*
Low power (10×)	Low	Partly open
High power (45×)	Midway	Half open
Oil-immersion	High	Fully open

Resolving Power of Objective

It is the ability of the objective to resolve each point on the minute object into widely spaced points, so that the points in the image can be seen as distinct and separate from one another, so as to get a clear un-blurred image.

It may appear that very high magnification can be obtained by using more number of high power lenses. Though possible, the highly magnified image obtained in this way is a blurred, one. That means, each point in the object cannot be found as widely spaced distinct and separate point on the image.

Mere increase in size (greater magnification) without the ability to distinguish structural details (greater resolution) is of little value. Therefore, the basic limitation in light microscopes is one not of magnification, but of resolving power, the ability to distinguish two adjacent points as distinct and separate, *i.e.* to resolve small components in the object into finer details on the image.

Resolving power is a function of two factors as given below

(a) Numerical aperture (n.a.)

(b) Wavelength of the light (λ)

(a) Numerical aperture

Numerical aperture is a numerical value concerned with the diameter of the objective lens in relation to its focal length. Thus, it is related to the size of the lower aperture of the objective, through which light enters into it. In a microscope, light is focused on the object as a narrow pencil of light, from where it enters into the objective as a diverging pencil The angle subtended by the optical axis (the line joining the centers of all the lenses) and the outermost ray still covered by the objective is a measure of the aperture called 'half aperture angle'.

A wide pencil of light passing through the object 'resolves' the points in the object into widely spaced points on the lens, so that the lens can produce these points as distinct and separate on the image. Here, the lens gathers more light.

On the other hand, a narrow pencil of light cannot 'resolve' the points in the object into widely spaced points on the lens, so that the lens produces a blurred image. Here, the lens gathers less light. Thus, the greater is the width of the pencil of light entering into the objective, the higher is its 'resolving power'

(b) Wavelength of the light (λ)

The smaller is the wavelength of light (λ), the greater is its ability to resolve the points on the object into distinctly visible finer details in the image. Thus, the smaller is the wavelength of light, the greater is its resolving power.

Working distance

The working distance of an objective is the distance between the front lens of the objective and the object slide when the image is in focus. Fig. 2.1: Working distance

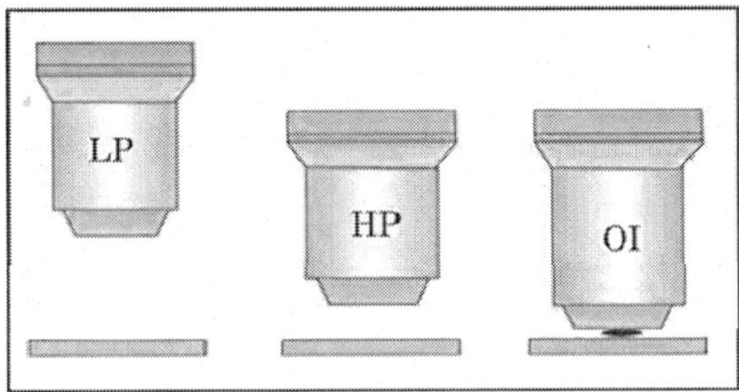

Fig. 2.1: Working distance

The greater the magnifying power of the objective, the smaller the working distance:

- × 10 objective: the working distance is 5–6 mm
- × 40 objective: the working distance is 0.5–1.5 mm
- × 100 objective: the working distance is 0.15–0.20 mm.

THE ADJUSTMENT SYSTEM

The adjusting system consists of two adjustments; the coarse adjustment and the fine adjustment. The coarse adjustment is used to obtain the approximate focus whereas the fine adjustment is used to obtain exact focus of the object after prior coarse adjustment.

Coarse Adjustment

It is a knob with rack and pinion mechanism to move the body tube up and down for focusing the object in the visible field. As rotation of the knob through a small angle moves the body tube through a long distance relative to the object, it can perform coarse adjustment. In modern microscopes, it moves the stage up and down and the body tube is fixed to the arm.

Fine Adjustment

It is a relatively smaller knob. Its rotation through a large angle can move the body tube only through a small vertical distance. It is used for fine adjustment to get the final clear image. In modern microscopes, fine adjustment is done by moving the stage up and down by the fine adjustment.

METHODS OF USE OF THE MICROSCOPE

Working Principle

The most commonly used microscope for general purposes is the standard compound microscope. It magnifies the size of the object by a complex system of lens arrangement.

It has a series of two lenses; (i) the objective lens close to the object to be observed and (ii) the ocular lens or eyepiece, through which the image is viewed by eye. Light from a light source (mirror or electric lamp) passes through a thin transparent object.

The objective lens produces a magnified 'real image' (first image) of the object. This image is again magnified by the ocular lens (eyepiece) to obtain a magnified 'virtual image' (final image), which can be seen by eye through the eyepiece. As light passes directly from the source to the eye through the two lenses, the field of vision is brightly illuminated. That is why; it is a bright-field microscope.

Procedure

The microscope should be handled carefully. Before using it examines the microscope, the student should follow the steps given below when using a compound microscope.

1. Place the microscope on the working table in the upright position and adjust the height and position of your chair so that you are comfortable and prepared for prolonged viewing. The eyepiece of the microscope should be level with and close to forearms on the table so that you can easily handle the adjustment screws. You need not remove your glasses if you use them constantly.
2. Check that the eyepiece and objectives are free from dust and oil. Use fresh lens tissue for this purpose.
3. Provide adequate illumination. If you have to use the external lamp, place it about 20 cm away from the microscope, switch on the lamp and allow the light to fall on the mirror. If you have to use natural light, place the microscope near the window for maximum illumination.
4. Select and adjust the mirror for optimal illumination according to the objective to be used. Direct the path of light to pass through the hole of the stage with maximum intensity while setting the mirror.

5. Place the slide with the object on the stage, so that it is held by the stage clips and pressed at the both ends in to close contact with the surface of the stage.
6. Make various microscopic adjustments to view the object under low-power objective

   The steps are:

   - Bring the low power objective (10X) into position by revolving the nosepiece
   - Adjust the illumination to improve contrast. Use the concave mirror, place the condenser at lowest position, and slightly open the iris.
   - Use the coarse focusing adjustment to focus the specimen on the slide
   - Use fine adjustment only to obtain and maintain exact focus. Put one hand one the focusing knob.
   - Bring the object of interest to the centre.
7. After preliminary screening under low power objective, proceed to examine the film under high power objective. The steps are:
   - Bring the high power objective (40X or 45X) into position by rotating the nosepiece; make sure that the objective clicks into place.
   - Use the concave mirror, raise the condenser slightly, and check the iris diaphragm is partially open so that illumination is properly centered. Increase the illumination as needed.
   - Repeat the procedure of focusing as described earlier by using the coarse adjustment knob in sequence.
8. After screening under the low power and examining high power, use the oil immersion objective to obtain greater details of the object.

   The steps are:

   - Swing away the high power objective and put a tiny drop of immersion oil on the slide over the path of light.

- Change the mirror to the plane side.
- Raise the condenser to maximum and open the iris fully to obtain maximum illumination.
- Turn the nosepiece and set the oil immersion objective in position; make sure that the objective has clicked into place.
- Use the fine adjustment knob to get the object in focus. If fails, look from the side, keep the eye level with the slide and lower the objective carefully with the coarse adjustment knob until the oil immersion objective touches the oil. Lower the objective further down and stop when the oil immersion objective touches the slide.

Precautions

1. Use only lens paper or Kimwipes to clean the optical parts of the microscope. Do not use paper towels, lab coat tails, handkerchiefs or other such to clean the lenses.
2. Never immerse the 10X or 40X lenses in oil.
3. When done each day, wipe off oil from the 100X oil immersion lens.
4. When done each day, clean stage, condenser lens, the other objective lenses and ocular lenses.

1. Do not attempt to clean the inside of the microscope or a lens.
2. Keep the microscope upright when taking or returning the microscope to the cabinet.
3. When the microscope is put away, the lowest power lens should be in place.

ROUTINE CARE AND MAINTENANCE OF THE MICROSCOPE

Transporting the Microscope

The compound light microscope is an expensive, precision instrument that must be handled appropriately. Demonstrate care in transporting, cleaning, using, and storing the microscope.

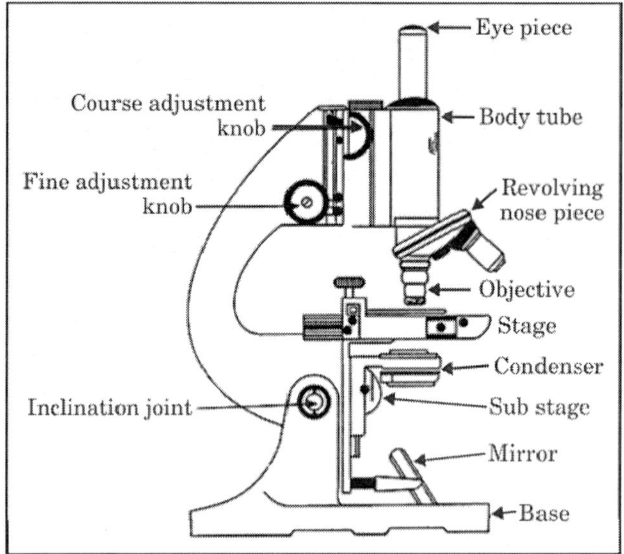

Fig. 2.2: Compound microscope and its parts

- Pick up the microscope with two hands, one holding the arm and the other.

  Supporting the base with the cord in a secure position.
- Carry the microscope upright so that a lens or eyepiece does not fall out, and carefully place the microscope on the lab table in front of you.

Maintenance of Microscopes

Microscope is costly equipment. Therefore, it should be handled carefully. Always keep the microscope in an upright position while taking it from one place to another. As far as possible don't tilt the arm. Clean the lenses of the microscope with the lens paper or muslin cloth, never with the filter or any other kind of paper. If you are using the high power objective lens then after the observation is over, turn the nose piece and bring low power objective lens in line with the hole in the stage. Objective lens should be kept at least 1 cm above the stage. After using the microscope always keep it in the box. Take care to see that the stage of microscope, the eye piece, the objective lens are dry and clean. No chemical should stick to these. Adjustment knobs and joints should be protected from rusting by applying vaseline.

Storing the Microscope

It is important to put the microscope away properly.

- Check that the scanning objective lens is in place and that the slide is removed from the stage.
- Depending on the type of microscope, either lower the stage or raise the objective to put maximum distance between the objective and the stage.
- Center the mechanical stage.
- Turn off the sub stage light. The bulb life is extended if it cools before moving the microscope.
- Clean the ocular and objective lenses with lens paper.
- Coil the cord neatly according to your instructor's directions.
- Place the dust cover over the microscope.
- Using both hands and the proper carrying technique, return the microscope to the appropriate cabinet.

Experiment No. 3

Aim: To Study Elementary Tissues

***Key words*:** Epithelial Tissue its Functions and Classification, Connective Tissue, Muscle Tissue, Nervous Tissue

Cells are highly organized units. But in multicultural organisms, they do not function in isolation. They work together in-group of similar cells called *tissue.* Tissue is a group of similar cell and their intercellular substance that have a similar embryological origin and function together to perform a specialized activity. A science that deals with the study of a tissue is Histology.

***There are four primary tissue types in the human body*:** Epithelial, connective, muscle, and nervous. *Epithelial tissue* covers surfaces, lines cavities, and forms glands. *Connective tissue*, the most abundant primary tissue in the body, connects different tissues, provides a framework, resists pulling forces, and protects other tissues. *Muscle tissue* causes movement, and *Nervous tissue* receives and generates nerve impulses. Organs are formed from two or more different tissues working together to perform a specific function.

EPITHELIAL TISSUE

Epithelial cells are arranged in continuous sheets, in single or multiple layers, Little intracellular space: cell junctions.

Epithelial cells have various surfaces which differ in structure and have specialised functions.

1) ***Apical (free) surface*:** Most superficial layer, faces the body surface, exposed to body cavity, lining of internal organ or exterior of body, and may contain cilia and microvilli.
2) ***Lateral surface*:** Face the adjacent cells on either side. May contain cell junctions (except hemidesmosomes).
3) ***Basal surface*:** Deepest layer, opposite to apical surface and adheres to extracellular material. Hemidesmosomes are present which anchor or attach the epithelial cells to a *basement membrane*.
4) ***Basement membrane*:** Thin extracellular layer made up of two layers.
   a) ***Basal lamina*:** Protein scaffolding secreted by epithelial cells. Contain proteins like collagen and laminin, glycoproteins and proteoglycans.
   b) ***Reticular lamina*:** (crossed collagen network) closer to underlying connective tissue and contains fibroblasts, which are the fibrous proteins produced by connective tissue cells that supports epithelium.

Functions of Epithelial Tissue

- ***Absorption*:** Certain epithelial cells lining the small intestine *absorb nutrients from the digestion of food*.
- ***Cleaning*:** Ciliated epithelium assists in *removing dust particles and foreign bodies* which have entered the air passages.
- ***Diffusion*:** Simple epithelium *promotes the diffusion of gases, liquids and nutrients*. Because they form such a thin lining, they are ideal for the diffusion of gases (*e.g.* walls of capillaries and lungs).
- ***Excretion*:** Epithelial tissues in the kidney *excrete waste products from the body and reabsorb needed materials from the urine*. *Sweat* is also excreted from the body by epithelial cells in the sweat glands.
- ***Protection*:** Epithelial cells from the skin *protect underlying tissue from mechanical injury, harmful chemicals, invading*

bacteria and from excessive loss of water.

- ***Reduces Friction*:** The smooth, tightly-interlocking, epithelial cells that line the entire circulatory system *reduce friction between the blood and the walls of the blood vessels.*
- ***Secretion*:** In glands, epithelial tissue is specialised to *secrete specific chemical substances* such as enzymes, hormones and lubricating fluids.
- ***Sensation*:** Sensory stimuli *penetrate specialised epithelial cells.* Specialised epithelial tissue containing sensory nerve endings is found in the skin, eyes, ears, nose and on the tongue.

Two Main Types

1) ***Covering and lining epithelium*:** Outer covering of the skin and lines some of the internal organs also *e.g.* blood vessels, ducts, body cavities and interior of the most important body systems.
2) ***Glandular epithelium*:** Constitutes secreting portion of glands *e.g.* thyroid gland, adrenal gland, sweat glands.

   - Classification of Covering and lining epithelium by considering both Arrangement of cells in layers and Shape of the cells:
   - ***Simple epithelium***

     1) *Simple squamous* (Table 3.1)

     2) *Simple cuboidal* (Table 3.2)

     3) *Simple columnar*

     a) Ciliated

     b) Non-ciliated (Table 3.3)
   - ***Stratified epithelium***

     1) *Stratified squamous*

     a) Keratinized

     b) Non-keratinized (Table 3.4)

     2) *Stratified cuboidal*

3) *Stratified columnar*

4) *Stratified transitional* (Table 3.5)

- ***Classification of Covering and lining epithelium*** by considering both arrangement of cells in layers and Shape of the cells.
- ***Pseudostratified columnar***

  a) Ciliated

  b) Non-ciliated (Table 3.6)

Microscopic Examination of Epithelia

1 Examine the photomicrograph of a simple squamous epithelium Fig. 3.1

- Observe how the epithelial cells fit close together to form a good barrier.
- Label the photomicrograph.

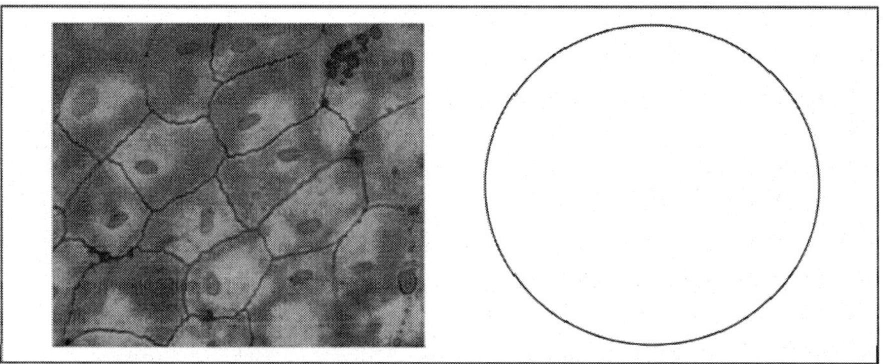

Fig. 3.1: Simple Squamous epithelium & Student drawing

2 Examine a microscope slide of a simple squamous epithelium. Use figure1 to help you locate the major structures. Draw the tissue in the space provided and label the major structures.

3 Stratified cuboidal and stratified columnar are not included because they are less common.

- On the survey photomicrograph (40X) for each tissue:
- Observe that the epithelial and connective tissue layers stain differently.
- Locate where the basement membrane forms the border between the epithelial and connective tissue layers.
- Note whether there is one epithelial cell layer (simple epithelium) or two or more epithelial cell layers (stratified epithelium).
- On the higher magnification photomicrograph (400 X) for each tissue:
- Examine the shape of the epithelial cell at the apical surface. This determines the tissue type as squamous, cuboidal, or columnar epithelium.
- Note any structural differences between apical surface and basal surface of epithelial tissue.
- Label the photomicrographs.

4 Review the location and function for each epithelial tissue type in Tables 1–6.

5 Examine prepared microscope slides showing tissue cross-sections. Use the survey photomicrographs in Figs. 6.3–6.9 to help you locate the epithelia at low power. Use the photomicrograph at 400_ to help you locate the major structures in each tissue. Draw each tissue in the space provided and label the major structures.

Table 3.1: Location and function of selected simple squamous epithelia

Location	*Function*
Mesothelium (epithelial layer of serous membranes)	Secretion of serous fluid into serous cavity.
alveoli (air sacs of lungs)	Single layer of squamous cells creates a short distance for *diffusion* of oxygen and carbon dioxide.
Glomerular capsule (part of filtration membrane in kidney)	Filtration of blood to form urine filtrate (substance that is converted into urine).
Endothelium of capillaries	Single layer of squamous cells creates a short distance for *diffusion* of substances between blood and interstitial fluid (tissue fluid).

Table 3.2: Location and function of selected simple cuboidal epithelia

Location	***Function***
Walls of kidney tubules	Modify urine filtrate by *absorption* of substances from the filtrate and *secretion* of other substances into the filtrate.
Glands	*Secretion* of products made by the simple cuboidal epithelial cells.

Table 3.3: Location and function of selected simple columnar epithelia

Location	***Function***
Lining of stomach and intestines	*Secretion* of digestive juices by simple columnar cells and secretion of mucus by goblet cells. In the small intestine the simple columnar epithelial cells have *microvilli* (*micro-* _ small; *villi* _ shaggy hair) to increase surface area for *absorption*.
Uterine tubes (Fallopian tubes)	Simple columnar epithelial cells have *cilia* that help *move* the egg to the uterus.
Central canal of spinal cord	Ciliated cells *move* cerebrospinal fluid.

Table 3.4: Location and function of selected stratified squamous epithelia

Location	***Function***
Surface of skin (keratinized stratified squamous epithelium)	Epithelial layer of skin is tough, dry,waterproof outer surface that forms a *protective barrier*
Lining of mouth, esophagus, anus, and vagina (nonkeratinized stratified squamous epithelium)	Moist epithelial layer that forms a *protective barrier* in areas subject to abrasion and friction

Table 3.5: Location and function of transitional epithelia

Location	***Function***
Lining of urinary bladder and parts of the ureters and the urethra	Provides a *protective barrier* that permits *distension.*

Table 3.6: Location and function of selected pseudostratified columnar epithelia

Location	***Function***
Lining of nasal cavity, trachea, and bronchi	*Secretion* of mucus by goblet cells. The columnar cells have *cilia* which *move* mucus toward the pharynx.

CONNECTIVE TISSUE

Connective tissue is the most abundant primary tissue in the body and has a variety of functions. It connects epithelial tissue to other tissues, forms the internal framework for soft organs, and forms tendons (connect muscle to bone) and ligaments (connect bone to bone).

Most abundant, widely distributed, and histologically variable of the 4 primary tissue types. Consists of cells that are typically widely separated by lots of extracellular material – referred to as the *extracellular matrix.* All connective tissues have the same embryonic origin - from mesodermal cells called mesenchyme.

Functions of Connective Tissue

- ***Binding of organs*:** Bones, tendons and ligaments
- ***Support*:** Bones, tendons and ligaments
- ***Physical protection*:** Bones and adipose tissue
- ***Immune protection*:** Blood and blood cells *e.g.* Phagocytes
- ***Movement*:** Bones, tendons and ligaments
- ***Storage*:** of energy and fat soluble substances
- Heat production and insulation

Classification of Connective Tissue

I. ***Embryonic connective tissue***

A. Mesenchyme

B. Mucous connective tissue

II. ***Mature connective tissue***

Fibrous connective tissue or connective tissue proper

A. *Loose connective tissue*

1. Areolar connective tissue
2. Adipose tissue
3. Reticular connective tissue

B. Dense connective tissue

1. Dense regular connective tissue
2. Dense irregular connective tissue
3. Elastic connective tissue

Supporting connective tissue

C. Cartilage

1. Hyline cartilage
2. Fibrocartilage
3. Elastic cartilage

D. Bone tissue

Fluid connective tissue

E. Blood tissue

F. Lymph

LOOSE CONNECTIVE TISSUE

Areolar Connective Tissue

Areolar connective tissue is loosely arranged, it is found wrapping organs and under skin, and holds and conveys tissue fluid. Contains primarily *fibroblasts*, but also macrophages, adipocytes and some blood cells. It contains all three fiber types, randomly arranged. The ground substance is fluid, semi-fluid or gelatinous. This tissue contains hyaluronic acid, which is thick and may slow the passage of some drugs. (Fig. 3.2) *Hylauronidase* is an enzyme produced by

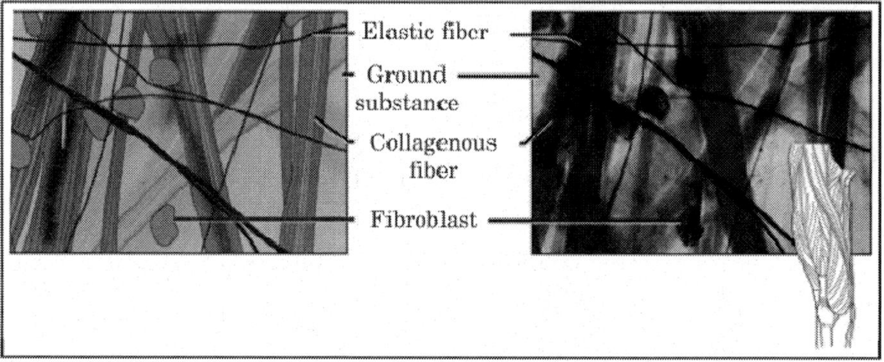

Fig. 3.2: Areolar connective tissue

WBC's, sperm and some bacteria. Injection of hyaluronidase can speed the passage of drugs and fluid through the tissue. Forms *subcutaneous layer* that attaches skin to underlying tissues and organs

Locations

- Underlying nearly all epithelia.
- Surrounding blood vessels, nerves, trachea, and esophagus.
- Between muscles.
- Within mesenteries, and the visceral layers of the pericardium and the pleura.

Functions

- Loosely binds epithelia to deeper tissues.
- Allows passage of nerves and blood vessels through other tissues.
- Provides an arena for immune defense.
- Blood vessels provide nutrients and waste removal for overlying epithelia.

Microscopic Appearance

- Loose arrangement of collagenous and elastic fibers. Some reticular fibers. (All 3 fiber types.)
- Scattered Cells. All 6 types can be present.
- Abundant ground substance.
- Numerous blood vessels. (Highly vascular.)

Adipose Tissue

Adipose tissue cells are adipocytes, and specialize in storing fat. Adipocytes are tightly packed, and very little matrix (Fig. 3.3). They accumulate under the skin and yellow marrow of long bones. Functions in energy reserves, insulation, protection, and support. Adults: white adipose tissue Newborns: brown adipose tissue (BAT).

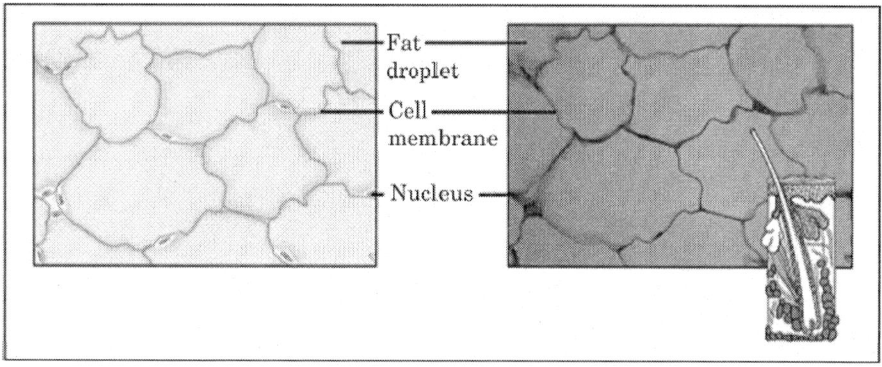

Fig. 3.3: Adipose tissue

Locations

- Subcutaneous fat beneath skin.
- Breast.
- Heart surface.
- *Cushioning organs*: Kidneys Eyes

Functions

- Energy storage.
- Thermal insulation.
- Shock absorption
- Protective cushioning for some organs.

Microscopic Appearance

- Dominated by adipocytes – large, empty-looking cells with thin margins.
- Nucleus usually pressed against the cell membrane – signet ring appearance.
- Often pale.
- Blood vessels often present.

Reticular Connective Tissue

Reticular connective tissue consists of reticular fibers and

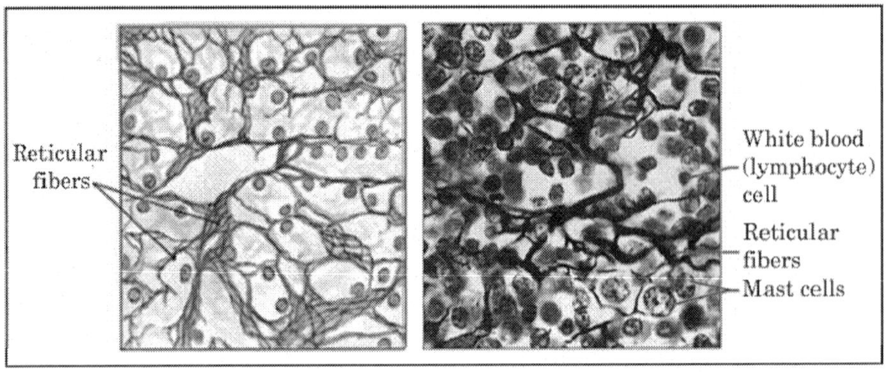

Fig. 3.4: Reticular connective tissue

fibroblasts and forms the supporting framework (stroma) for cells in the liver, spleen, lymph nodes and bone marrow. (Fig. 3.4).

Locations

- Lymph nodes, spleen, thymus, and bone marrow.

Functions

- The branching network of reticular fibers will form a scaffold-like framework (stroma) for lymphatic organs. *e.g.* Spleen, thymus, and lymph nodes.
- Binds smooth muscle together
- Reticular fibers in spleen filter blood and remove worn-out cells
- Reticular fibers in lymph nodes filter lymph and removes bacteria

Microscopic Appearance

- Loose network of reticular fibers and a type of fibroblast known as the reticular cell.
- Infiltrated with numerous white blood cells.
- Often appears dark purple or black.

DENSE CONNECTIVE TISSUE

Dense Regular Connective Tissue

Dense regular connective tissue collagen fibers are arranged in parallel bundles which makes this tissue flexible, but resistant to stretching. Fibroblasts are found in rows between the fibers. Found in tendons and ligaments. Blood supply is poor. (Fig. 3.5).

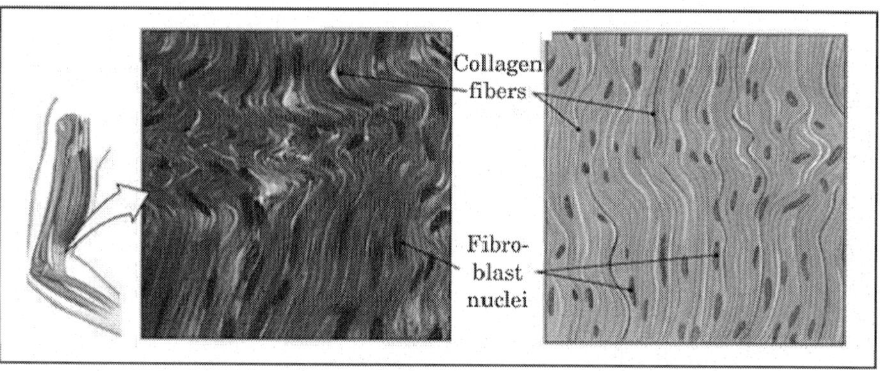

Fig. 3.5: Dense regular connective tissue

Locations

- Tendons and Ligaments

Functions

- Ligaments bind bone tightly to other bones.
- Resist stress.
- Tendons attach skeletal muscles to bone and transfer muscular tension to bones.

Microscopic Appearance

- Densely packed, parallel, often wavy collagenous fibers.
- Slender fibroblast nuclei compressed between bundles of collagenous fibers.
- Scanty open space (little ground substance)
- Scarcity of blood vessels

Dense Irregular Connective Tissue

Also has collagen fibers and fibroblasts, but the collagen fibers are thicker and arranged irregularly. This tissue usually forms sheets, and resists pulling in many directions. It is found in heart valves, around cartilage, bone, muscles, dermis of skin, and around some organs. (Fig. 3.6).

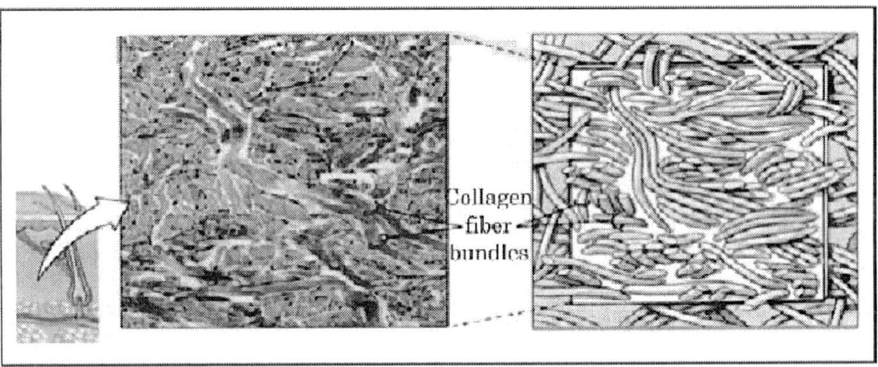

Fig. 3.6: Dense irregular connective tissue

Locations

- Deeper portion of dermis of skin.
- Capsules around visceral organs such as the liver, spleen, and kidneys.
- Fibrous sheaths around cartilages and bones.

Functions

- Provides a durable, hard to tear structure that can withstand stresses placed in unpredictable directions.

Microscopic Appearance

- Densely packed, collagenous fibers running in random directions. Compare this to dense regular CT.
- Scanty open space
- Few visible cells.
- Scarcity of blood vessels.

Elastic Connective Tissue

Consists of elastic fibers (giving yellowish colour) and fibroblasts. Very elastic. It is found in the lungs, walls of arteries, bronchial tubes and in the attachments between the vertebrae. Strong and can regain its original shape after being stretched (Fig. 3.7).

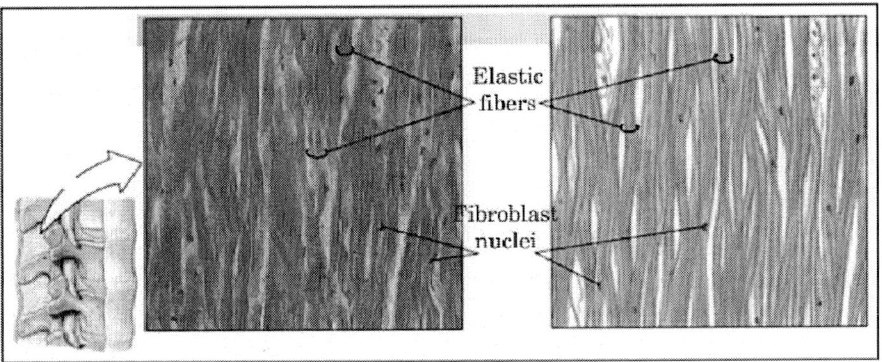

Fig. 3.7: Elastic connective tissue

Location

- Between vertebrae of the spinal column (Ligamentum flavum and ligamentum nuchae); ligaments supporting penis; ligaments supporting transitional epithelia; in blood vessel walls.

Function

- Stablilzes position of vertebrae and penis; cushions shocks; permits expansion and contraction of organs.

Cartilage

Cartilage has a dense network of collagen fibers, which gives strength, and elastic fibers. The matrix contains chondroitin sulfate, which is rubbery and gives cartilage resilience (ability to assume original shape after deformation). Cells are chondrocytes, and are found in lacuanae. Surface of cartilage is surrounded by perichondrium, where blood vessels are located. No blood supply in the cartilage itself.

Hyaline Cartilage (Fig. 3.8)

- Most abundant cartilage.
- It has very fine collagen fibers and a resilient gel as its ground substance.
- Found in: embryonic skeleton, at the ends of bones, in the nose, and in respiratory structures.
- It is flexible, allows movement, reduces friction, absorbs shock and provides support. Important in bone growth and repair.

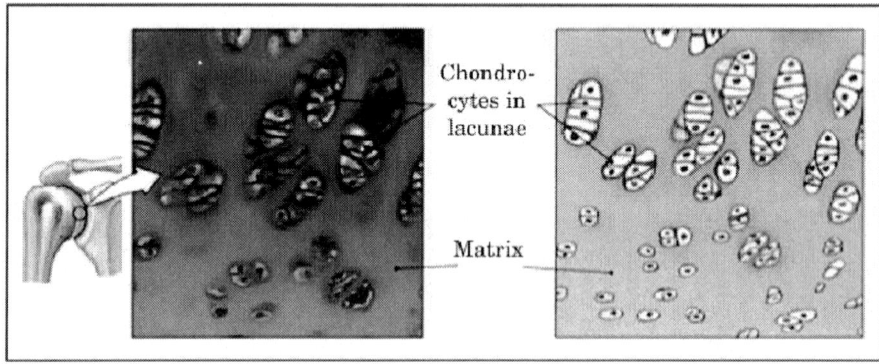

Fig. 3.8: Hyaline cartilage

Locations

- Forms the majority of the fetal skeleton.
- Forms boxlike structure around larynx and supportive rings around trachea and bronchi.
- Attaches ribs to the sternum.
- Forms a thin *articular cartilage* over the ends of bones at moveable joints.

Functions

- Eases joint movements.
- Keeps airways patent.
- Moves vocal cords.

- Precursor of bone in the fetal skeleton.
- Structural attachment

Microscopic Appearance

- Clear, glassy matrix, often stained light blue or pink.
- *Hyalos* is Greek for glass.
- Fine, dispersed collagenous fibers, not usually visible.
- Chondrocytes often in small clusters of 3-4 cells within a single lacuna (known as cell nests or isogenous groups).
- Covered by a perichondrium – a fibrous sheath made of dense irregular connective tissue.

Fibrocarilage (Fig. 3.9)

Locations

- Pubic symphysis – the anterior joint between the 2 halves of the pelvic girdle.
- Intervertebral discs that separate the bones of the spinal column.
- Menisci (shock-absorbing pads of cartilage) in the knee joint.
- At points where tendons insert on bones near articular hyaline cartilage.

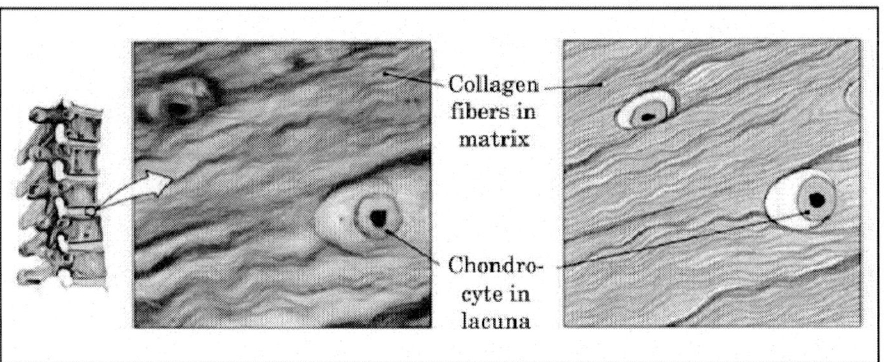

Fig. 3.9: Fibrocartilage

Functions

- Resists compression and absorbs shock in some joints.
- Often a transitional structure between dense connective tissue and hyaline cartilage.
- For example, at some tendon-bone junctions.

Elastic Cartilage

Has condrocytes in a network of elastic fibers. It maintains the shape of organs such as the epiglottis of the larynx, auditory (Eustachian) tubes, and external ear. (Fig. 3.10).

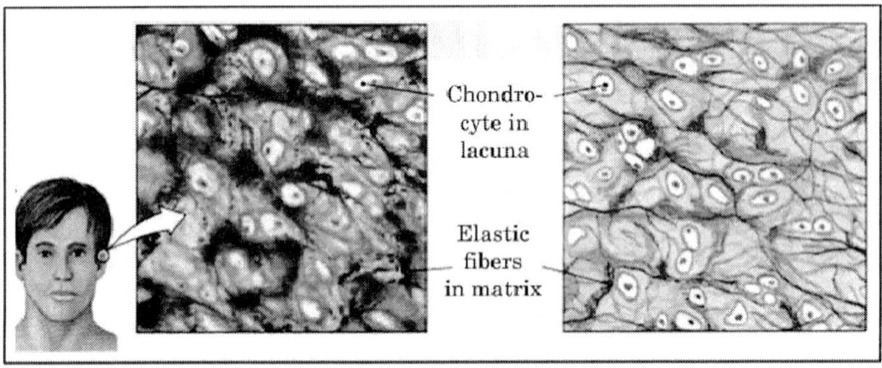

Fig. 3.10: Elastic cartilage

Locations

- Epiglottis – flap of tissue that covers the tracheas when you swallow to prevent food/liquid from going down the "wrong pipe."
- Eustachian tube – connects the ear to the nasopharynx

Function

- Provides flexible, elastic support

Microscopic Appearance

- Elastic fibers form web-like mesh amid lacunae.
- Always covered by a perichondrium.

Bone Tissue

(Osseous tissue) consists of collagen fibers (flexibility), mineral salts (that contribute to the hardness of bone) and cells called osteocytes. It is covered by the *periosteum* and lined by the *endosteum*. It can be *compact* or *spongy* depending on how the matrix and the cells are organized. The basic unit of compact bone is the *osteon* or *Haversian system*. (Fig. 3.11).

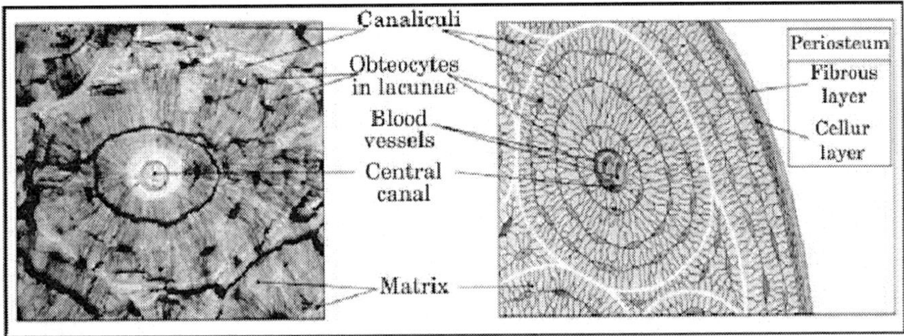

Fig. 3.11: Bone tissue

It supports, protects, helps provide movement, stores minerals, and houses blood-forming tissue. Each osteon has four parts:

1. Lamellae (little plates): Concentric rings of matrix containing mineral salts (Ca and PO_4) responsible for bone hardness and collagen fibers that give bone strength. Lamellae give compact nature to bones
2. Lacunae are small spaces between lamellae and contains osteocytes
3. Canaliculi network of minute canals containing the processes of osteocytes. They also provide routes for nutrients to reach osteocytes and for wastes to leave them
4. Central canal (Haversian) contains blood vessels and
5. *Spongy bones* lacks osteon. But they consists of columns of bones known as *trabeculae* containing lacunae and canaliculi. Spaces between lacunae are filled with red bone marrow.

Blood Tissue

It consists of plasma and formed elements (erythrocytes, leukocytes, and platelets). Functionally, its cells transport oxygen and carbon dioxide, carry on phagocytosis, participate in allergic reactions, provide immunity, and bring about blood clotting.

Lymph Tissue

Extracellular fluid flowing in lymphatic vessels. It consists of clear fluid similar to blood plasma but contains less proportion of proteins. It is also full of cells and chemicals and composition depends on the type of the organs. *e.g.* lymph from lymph nodes and that of small intestine.

MUSCLE TISSUE

Muscle tissue is very cellular, with most of the tissue consisting of muscle cells. All muscle tissues are highly vascularized and are innervated. Muscle cells are elongated cells called *fibers* that shorten (contract) when stimulated, causing movement. There are three types of muscle tissue—skeletal, cardiac, and smooth—with each type having a distinct appearance.

- Muscle tissue consists of elongated cells known as muscle fibers.
- Muscle fibers use ATP to generate force which helps muscle tissue to carryout various functions *e.g.* body movements, posture and heat generation.

These tissues are classified into three types depending upon their location, structure and function.

1. Skeletal muscle tissue
2. Cardiac muscle tissue
3. Smooth muscle tissue

Functions

- Body movement

- Maintenance of posture
- Respiration
- Production of body heat
- Communication
- Constriction of organs and vessels
- Heart beat

Skeletal Muscle Tissue (Fig. 3.12)

- They are named so because of their location.
- Usually attached to and cover the bony skeleton.
- It is striated: *i.e.* they contain alternate light and dark bands called as *striations* which can be visualised under light microscope.
- It is controlled *voluntarily i.e.* it can be made to Contract or Relax by conscious control.
- *Skeletal muscles* are responsible for all locomotion, posture, joint stabilization and heat generation

Location

Skeletal muscle tissue is organized by connective tissues into the skeletal muscles.

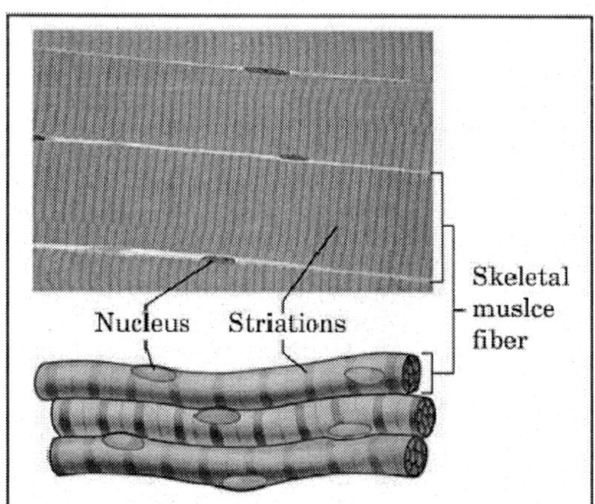

Fig. 3.12: Skeletal muscle

Functions

Skeletal muscle tissue functions in the

(1) Production of voluntary body movements and
(2) Heat production.

Cardiac Muscle Tissue (Fig. 3.13)

- Forms most of the wall of heart.
- It is striated but involuntary type of muscle.
- Cardiac muscle fibers are branched and usually have only one centrally located nucleus.
- Muscle cells are attached end to end by intercalated discs which are unique to cardiac muscles.
- Intercalated discs contain desmosomes and gap junctions

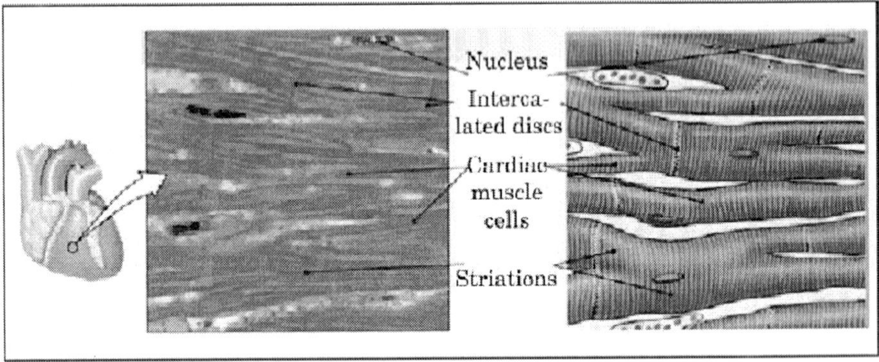

Fig. 3.13: Cardiac muscle

Location

Cardiac muscle for the muscle of the heart.

Function

The muscle of the heat functions in producing the heart's involuntary contractions.

Bone Tissue

Smooth Muscle Tissue

Located in the walls of hollow internal structures *e.g.* blood vessels, stomach, intestine, airways to lungs, urinary bladder etc. (Fig. 3.14).

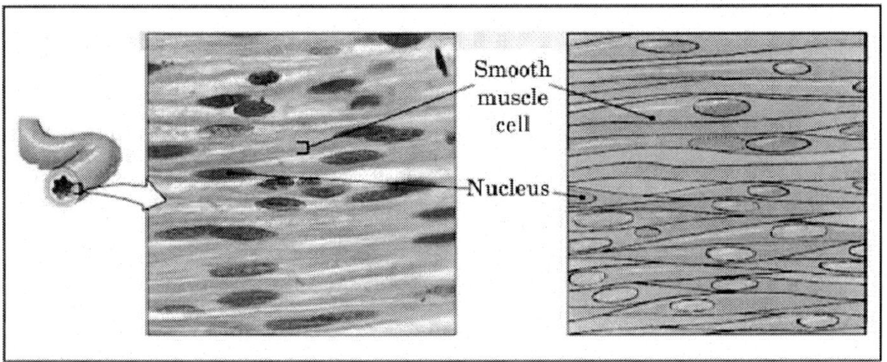

Fig. 3.14: Smooth muscle

Structure

Smooth muscle is organized into muscular sheets that surround or enclose many of the body's hollow organs. Its fibres are characterized by being

(1) Long,
(2) Spindle shaped
(3) Uninucleate, and
(4) Nonstriated (smooth)

Locations

Smooth muscle is located in the walls of many of the hollow organs such as the

(1) Esophagus,
(2) Stomach,
(3) Intestines,

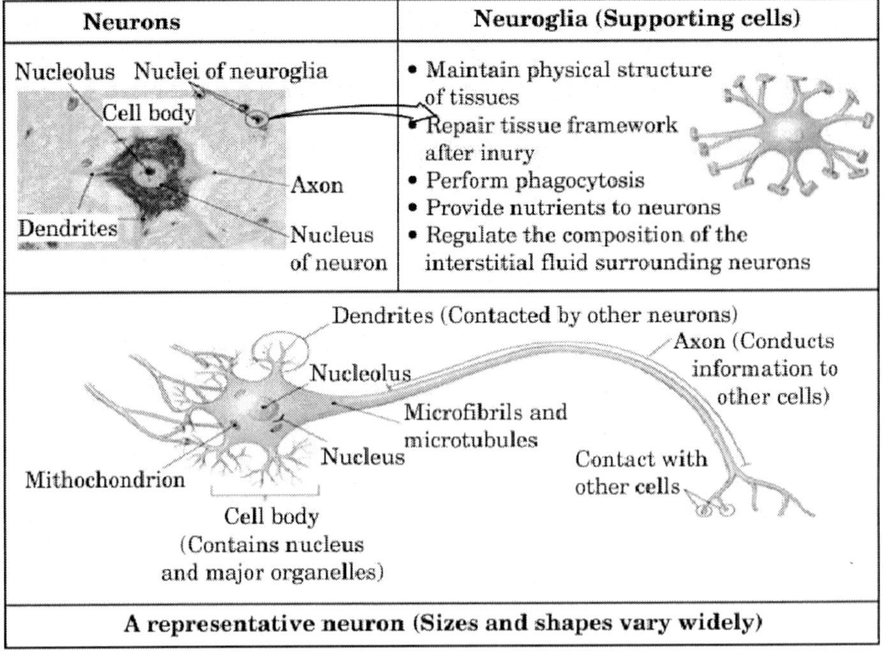

Fig. 3.15: Nervous tissue

(4) Urinary bladder, and
(5) Blood vessels.

Functions

Smooth muscle functions in producing *involuntary contractions* that move materials through the organs it surrounds.

Smooth muscle has great plasticity; it can undergo considerable stretching without appreciably reducing its ability to contract.

NERVOUS TISSUE

Nervous tissue, which forms the brain, spinal cord, and nerves, is very cellular. Two basic categories of nervous tissue cells are *neurons* and *neuroglia* (*neuro* _ nerve; *glia* _ glue). Neurons receive and send information, whereas neuroglia support the neurons and help them to function. Neurons have one or more processes (cellular extensions) that receive or send information as nerve impulses. *Dendrites* (*dendro* _ tree) are processes that receive signals from sensory receptors or other neurons. An *axon* is a process that sends signals to other neurons, muscles, or glands. Neurons have one axon but may have many dendrites. The main part of the cell where the nucleus is located is called the *cell body*. (Fig. 3.15) In the following activity you will observe only ultipolar *neurons*, which are neurons with many processes.

Experiment No. 4

Aim: To Study Human Skeleton

Key words: Osteology, Division of skeleton, Structure of bone, Histology of bone, Types of bone, Bone markings,

Human skeletal system is the system of bones, associated cartilages and joints of human body.

Osteology is the study of the human skeleton, which includes all bones of the body. It is important to know the correct descriptive terminology when speaking of the various bones and regions, *i.e.*, the bone of the upper leg is the femur, not the thigh-bone.

Skeleton is defined as the hard framework of human body around which the entire body is built. Almost all the hard parts of human body are components of human skeletal system. Joints are very important because they help the skeleton system to move at different locations.

Bone is living tissue, and, as such, can grow and remodel during a person's lifetime. The three types of bone cells are the osteoblasts, which are responsible for bone growth; the osteoclasts, which are active in bone resorption; and the osteocytes, which serve a regulatory function, adjusting the circulating levels of bone minerals. Because bone is malleable, it can be modified through exercise, disease, injury, and diet.

Divisions of Skeleton

The average adult skeleton has 206 bones (Fig. 4.1, Fig. 4.2). Although this is the traditional number, the actual number of bones varies from person to person and decreases with age as some bones become fused. Bones can be categorized as paired or unpaired. A *paired bone* is two bones of the same type located on the right and left sides of the body, whereas an *unpaired bone* is a bone located on the midline of the body. For example, the bones of the upper and lower limbs are paired bones, whereas the bones of the vertebral column are unpaired bones. There are 86 paired and 34 unpaired bones.

The skeleton is divided into the axial and appendicular skeletons.

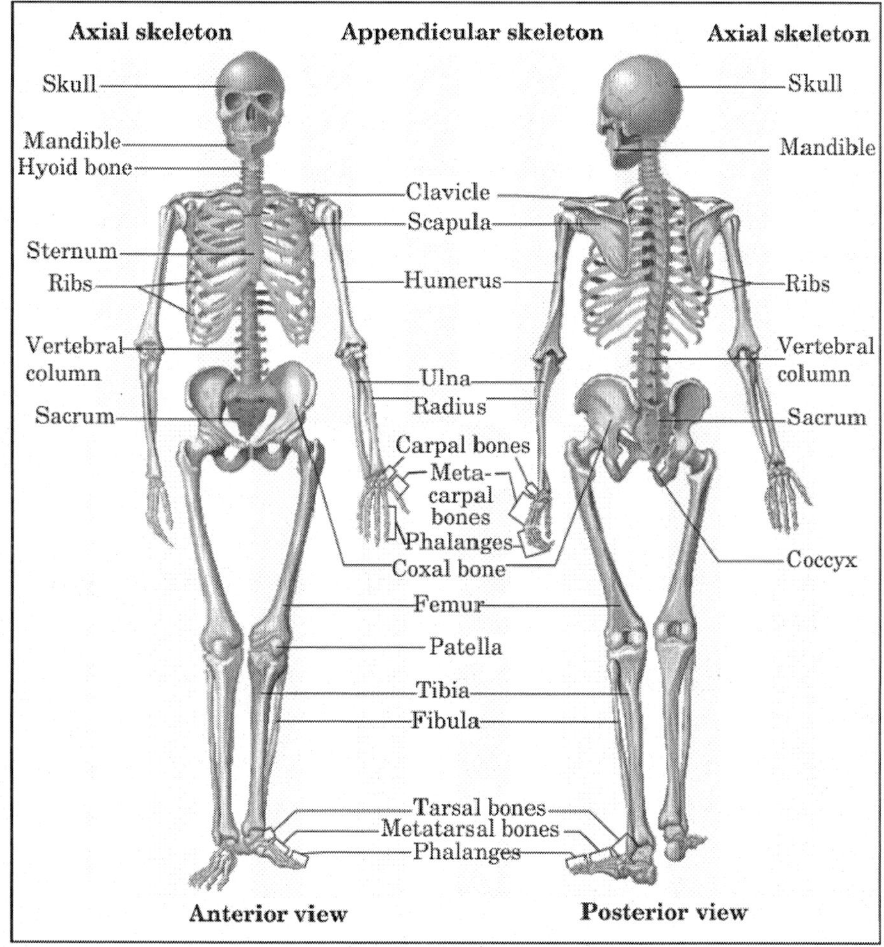

Fig. 4.1: Complete skeleton

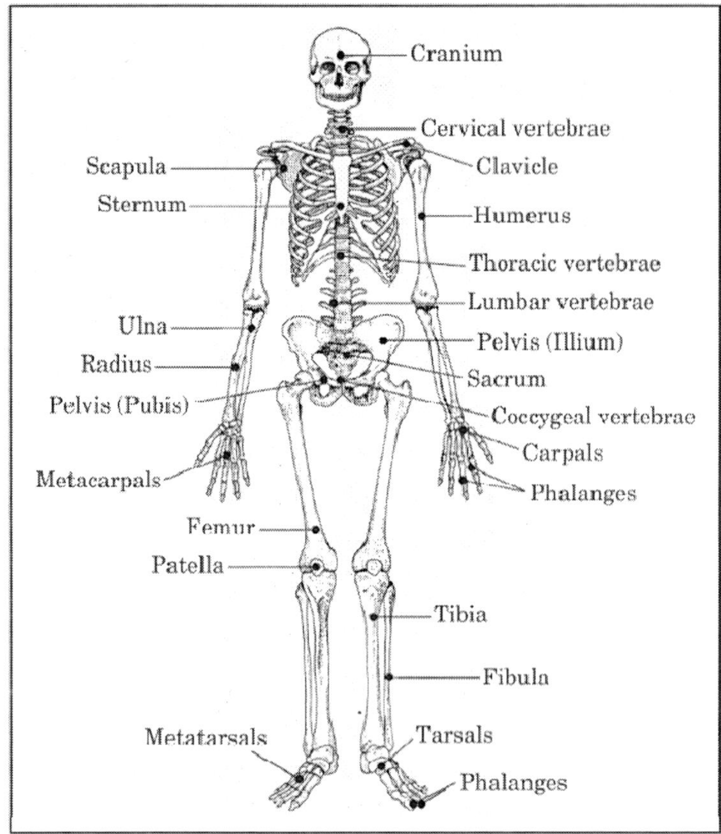

Fig. 4.2: Complete skeleton

Bones of the axial skeleton are listed in the far left- and right-hand columns; bones of the appendicular skeleton are listed in the center. (The skeleton is not shown in the anatomical position).

Bones of the axial skeleton are listed in the far left- and right-hand columns; bones of the appendicular skeleton are listed in the center. (The skeleton is not shown in the anatomical position.)

AXIAL SKELETON

The *axial skeleton* forms the upright axis of the body (Fig. 4.1). It is divided into the skull, auditory ossicles, hyoid bone, vertebral column, and thoracic cage, or rib cage. The axial skeleton protects the brain, the spinal cord, and the vital organs housed within the thorax. The 22 bones of the skull are divided into two groups: those of the braincase and those of the face. The *braincase* consists of 8 bones that immediately surround and protect the brain.

SKULL

The bones of the head form the *skull*, or *cranium.*

- 1 Frontal bone
- 2 Parietal bones
- 2 Temporal bones
- 1 Tccipital bone
- 1 Sphenoid bone
- 1 Ethmoid bone

The *facial bones* form the structure of the face. The facial bones support the organs of vision, smell, and taste. They also provide attachment points for the muscles involved in *mastication* (chewing), facial expression, and eye movement. The jaws (mandible and maxillae) hold the teeth and the temporal bones hold the *auditory ossicles,* or ear bones. The bones of the skull, except for the mandible, are not easily separated from each other. It is convenient to think of the skull, except for the mandible, as a single unit. The top of the skull is called the *calvaria* or skullcap. It is usually cut off to reveal the skull's interior.

- 2 Zygomatic or cheek bones
- 1 Maxilla (originated as 2)
- 2 Nasal bones
- 2 Lacrimal bones
- 1 Vomer
- 2 Palatine bones
- 2 Inferior conchae
- 1 Mandible (originated as 2)

APPENDICULAR SKELETON

The appendicular skeleton (see figure 1) consists of the bones of the *upper* and *lower limbs* and the *girdles* by which they are attached to the body. The term *girdle* means a belt or a zone and refers to the two zones, pectoral and pelvic, where the limbs are attached to the body. The pectoral girdle attaches the upper limbs to the body and allows considerable movement of the upper limbs. This freedom of movement allows the hands to be placed in a wide range of positions to accomplish their functions. The pelvic girdle attaches the lower limbs to the body, providing support while allowing movement. The pelvic girdle is stronger and attached much more firmly to the body than is the pectoral girdle, and the lower limb bones in general are thicker and longer than those of the upper limb.

Pectoral Girdle or Shoulder Girdle

Each shoulder girdle consists of:

- 1 Clavicle
- 1 Scapula.

Each upper limb consists of the following bones:

- 1 Humerus
- 1 Radius
- 1 Ulna
- 8 Carpal bones
- 5 Metacarpal bones
- 14 Phalanges.

Pelvic Girdle

The bones of the pelvic girdle consist of two innominate bones and one sacrum.

The bones of the pelvic girdle are:

- 2 Innominate bones
- 1 Sacrum.

The bones of the lower limb are:

- 1 Femur • 7 Tarsal bones
- 1 Tibia • 5 Metatarsal bones
- 1 Fibula • 14 Phalanges.
- 1 Patella

Structure of Bone

General structure of a long bone: These have a *diaphysis* or shaft and two *epiphyses* or extremities. The diaphysis is composed of *compact bone* with a central medullary canal, containing fatty *yellow bone marrow.* The epiphyses consist of an outer covering of compact bone with *cancellous bone* inside. The diaphysis and epiphyses are separated by *epiphyseal cartilages,* which ossify when growth is complete. Thickening of a bone occurs by the deposition of new bone tissue under the periosteum. Long bones are almost completely covered by a vascular membrane, the *periosteum.* The outer layer is fibrous and the inner layer is osteogenic containing *osteoblasts* (bone-forming cells) and *osteoclasts* (bone-destroying cells), which are involved in maintenance and remodeling of bones; it gives attachment to muscles and tendons and protects bones from injury. *Hyaline cartilage* replaces periosteum on the articular surfaces of bones forming synovial joints.

Structure of Short, Irregular, Flat and Sesamoid Bones

These have a relatively thin outer layer of compact bone with cancellous bone inside containing *red bone marrow* (Fig. 4.3). They are enclosed by periosteum except the inner layer of the cranial bones where it is replaced by dura mater.

HISTOLOGY OF BONE

Bone cells

The cells responsible for bone formation are *osteoblasts* (these later mature into *osteocytes*). Osteoblasts and *chondrocytes* (cartilage-

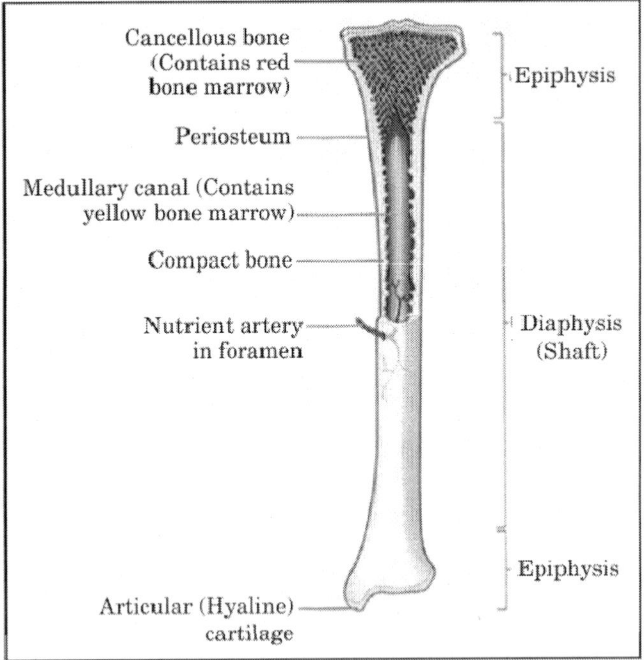

Fig. 4.3: A mature long bone

forming cells) develop from the same parent fibrous tissue cells. Differentiation into *osteogenic cells,* rather than *chondroblasts,* is believed to depend upon an adequate oxygen supply. This may be a factor affecting healing of fractures, *i.e.* if the oxygen supply is deficient there may be a preponderance of chondroblasts, resulting in a cartilaginous union of the fracture.

Osteoblasts

These are the bone-forming cells that secrete collagen and other constituents of bone tissue. They are present:

- In the deeper layers of periosteum
- In the centres of ossification of immature bone
- At the ends of the diaphysis adjacent to the epiphyseal cartilages of long bones
- At the site of a fracture.

Osteocytes

As bone develops, osteoblasts become trapped and remain isolated in lacunae. They stop forming new bone at this stage and are called *osteocytes.* Osteocytes are nourished by tissue fluid in the canaliculi that radiate from the Haversian canals. Their functions are not clear but they may be associated with the movement of calcium between the bones and the blood.

Osteoclasts

Their function is resorption of bone to maintain the optimum shape. This takes place at bone surfaces:

- Under the periosteum, to maintain the shape of bones during growth and to remove excess callus formed during healing of fractures
- Round the walls of the medullary canal during growth and to canalise callus during healing.

TYPES OF BONE

1. **Long Bones**—The bones of the arms, legs, hands, and feet (but not the wrists and ankles). The shaft of a long bone is the *diaphysis*, and the ends are called *epiphyses*. The diaphysis is made of compact bone and is hollow, forming a canal within the shaft. This *arrow canal* (or medullary cavity) contains *yellow bone marrow*, which is mostly adipose tissue. The epiphyses are made of spongy bone covered with a thin layer of compact bone. Although red bone marrow is present in the epiphyses of children's bones, it is largely replaced by yellow bone marrow in adult bones.
2. **Short Bones**—The bones of the wrists and ankles.
3. **Flat Bones**—The ribs, shoulder blades, hip bones, and cranial bones.
4. **Irregular Bones**—The vertebrae and facial bones.

Short, flat, and irregular bones are all made of spongy bone covered with a thin layer of compact bone. Red bone marrow is found within the spongy bone. The joint surfaces of bones are covered with *articular cartilage*, which provides a smooth surface. Covering the rest of the bone is the *periosteum,* a fibrous connective tissue membrane whose collagen fibers merge with those of the tendons and ligaments that are attached to the bone. The periosteum anchors these structures and contains both the blood vessels that enter the bone itself and osteoblasts that will become active if the bone is damaged.

Bone Markings

Most bones have rough surfaces, raised protuberances and ridges which give attachment to muscle tendons and ligaments. These are not included in the following descriptions of individual bones unless they are of particular note, but many are marked on illustrations. (Table 4.1).

Table 4.1: Bone markings

Term	*Description*	*Examples*
Angle	An inside or outside corner	Angle of mandible Lateral angle of scapula
Aperture	Opening on surface of space within a bone	Nasal aperture
Body	The main or central portion	Body of sphenoid bone Body of vertebra of a bone
Border	Edge or boundary of a bone	Superior border of scapula Medial border of scapula
Capitulum	A small articular swelling	Capitulum near head of rib
Condyle	Rounded bump; usually fits into a fossa on another bone to form a joint	Occipital condyle Lateral condyle of femur
Crest	Moderately raised ridge; generally a site for muscle attachment	Iliac crest of pelvic bone Pubic crest of pelvic bone
Epicondyle	Bump near a condyle; often gives the appearance of a "bump on a bump"; for muscle attachment	Lateral epicondyle of humerus Lateral epicondyle of femur
Facet	Flat surface that forms a joint with another facet or flat bone	Superior articular facet of vertebra Inferior articular facet of vertebra
Fissure	Long, cracklike hole for blood vessels / nerves	Superior orbital fissure of sphenoid Inferior orbital fissure of sphenoid

Table 4.1: (*Contd...*)

Table 4.1: (*Contd...*)

Term	*Description*	*Examples*
Foramen	Round hole for vessels and nerves	Stylomastoid foramen of temporal bone Jugular foramen of temporal Bone
Fossa	Depression; often receives an articulating bone	Mandibular fossa of temporal bone Jugular fossa of temporal bone
Head	Distinct epiphysis on a long bone, separated from the shaft by a narrowed portion	Head of rib Head of humerus
Line	Similar to a crest but not raised as much	Superior nuchal line of occipital bone Inferior nuchal line of occipital bone
Margin	Edge of a flat bone or flat area	Supraorbital margin of frontal bone Infraorbital margin of maxilla
Meatus	Tubelike opening or channel	External acoustic meatus of temporal bone. Internal acoustic meatus of temporal bone
Neck	A narrowed portion, usually at the base of a head	Neck of mandible Anatomical neck of humerus
Notch	A V-like "cut" out of the margin or edge of a flat area	Supraorbital notch Radial notch of ulna
Process	Projection or raised area	Mastoid process of temporal bone Spinous process of vertebra
Ramus	Curved portion of a bone, like a ram's horn	Ramus of mandible Superior pubic ramus
Sinus	Cavity within a bone	Frontal sinus Ethmoid sinus
Spine	Sharp, pointed process; simi-ilar to crested but raised more; for muscle attachment	Spine of scapula Anterior superior spine
Sulcus	Groove or elongated depression	Intertubercular sulcus Radial sulcus
Trochanter	Large bump for muscle attachment	Greater trochanter of femur Lesser trochanter of femur
Tubercle	Small tuberosity	Tubercle of rib Pubic tubercle
Tuberosity	Oblong, raised bump, usually for muscle attachment; also called a *tuber*; a small tube rosity is called a *tubercle*	Frontal tuberosity Deltoid tuberosity of humerus

FUNCTIONS OF BONE

Bones have a variety of functions. They:

- Provide the framework of the body
- Give attachment to muscles and tendons

- Permit movement of the body as a whole and of parts of the body, by forming joints that are moved by muscles
- Form the boundaries of the cranial, thoracic and pelvic cavities, protecting the organs they contain
- Contain red bone marrow in which blood cells develop: haematopoiesis
- Provide a reservoir of minerals, especially calcium phosphate.

FUNCTIONS OF SKELETON

The skeleton system serves 6 major functions to human body.

1. ***Support***: The skeleton provides the framework which supports the body and maintains its shape. The pelvis and associated ligaments and muscles provide a floor for the pelvic structures. Without the ribs, costal cartilages and the inter-costal muscles the heart would collapse.
2. ***Movement***: The joints between bones permit movement, some allowing a wider range of movement than others, *e.g.* the ball and socket joint allows a greater range of movement than the pivot joint at the neck. Movement is powered by skeletal muscles, which are attached to the skeleton at various sites on bones. Muscles, bones, and joints provide the principal mechanics for movement, all co-ordinate by the nervous system.
3. ***Protection***: The skeleton protects many vital organs like, the skull protects the brain, eyes, and the middle and inner ears, the vertebrae protects the spinal cord, the rib cage, spine, and sternum protect the lungs, heart and major blood vessels, the clavicle and scapula protect the shoulder, the ilium and spine protect the digestive and urogenital systems and the hip, the patella and the ulna protect the knee and the elbow respectively, the carpals and tarsals protect the wrist and ankle respectively.
4. ***Blood Cell Production***: The skeleton is the site of haematopoiesis, which takes place in red bone marrow.
5. ***Storage***: Bone matrix can store calcium and is involved in calcium metabolism, and bone marrow can store iron in

ferritin and is involved in iron metabolism. However, bones are not entirely made of calcium, but a mixture of chondroitin sulfate and hydroxyapatite, the latter making up 70% of a bone.

6. ***Endocrine Regulation*:** Bone cells release a hormone called osteocalcin, which contributes to the regulation of blood sugar (glucose) and fat deposition. Osteocalcin increases both the insulin secretion and sensitivity, in addition to boosting the number of insulin-producing cells and reducing fat storage.

Experiment No. 5

AIM: To Study the Bones of Skull and Thorax

***Key words*:** Cranial bones, Facial bones, Thoracic cage and Ribs

INTRODUCTION

***Skull*:** The skull rests on the upper end of the vertebral column and its bony structure is divided into two parts: the cranium and the face. (Table 5.1).

CRANIAL BONES

The cranium is formed by a number of flat and irregular bones that provide a bony protection for the brain (Fig. 5.1). It has a *base* upon which the brain rests and a *vault* that surrounds and covers it. The periosteum inside the skull bones consists of the outer layer of dura mater. In the mature skull the joints *(sutures)* between the bones are immovable (fibrous). The bones have mumerous perforations (*e.g.* foramina, fissures) through which nerves, blood and lymph vessels pass. The bones of the cranium are:

1 Frontal bone
2 Parietal bones
2 Temporal bones
1 Occipital bone
1 Sphenoid bone
2 Ethmoid bone

Table 5.1: Bones of the Skull—Important parts

Bone	***Part***	***Description***
Frontal	• Frontal sinus • Coronal suture	• Air cavity that opens into nasal cavity • Joint between frontal and parietal bones
Parietal (2)	• Sagittal suture	• Joint between the 2 parietal bones
Temporal (2)	• Squamosal suture • External auditory meatus • Mastoid process • Mastoid sinus • Mandibular fossa • Zygomatic process	• Joint between temporal and parietal bone • The tunnel-like ear canal • Oval projection behind the ear canal • Air cavity that opens into middle ear • Oval depression anterior to the ear canal; articulates with mandible • Anterior projection that articulates with the zygomatic bone
Occipital	• Foramen magnum • Condyles	• Large opening for the spinal cord • Oval projections on either side of the foramen magnum; articulate with the atlas
Sphenoid	• Lambdoidal suture • Greater wing • Sella turcica	• Joint between occipital and parietal bones • Flat, lateral portion between the frontal and temporal bones • Central depression that encloses the pituitary Gland
Ethmoid	• Sphenoid sinus • Ethmoid sinus • Crista galli • Cribriform plate & olfactory foramina • Perpendicular plate • Conchae (4 are part of ethmoid; 2 inferior)	• Air cavity that opens into nasal cavity • Air cavity that opens into nasal cavity • Superior projection for attachment of meninges • On either side of base of crista galli ol factory nerves pass through foramina • Upper part of nasal septum • Shelf-like projections into nasal cavities that 'increase surface area of nasal mucosa are separate bones
Mandible	• Body • Condyles • Sockets	• U-shaped portion with lower teeth • Oval projections that articulate with the temporal bones • Conical depressions that hold roots of lower Teeth
Maxilla (2)	• Maxillary sinus • Palatine process • Sockets	• Air cavity that opens into nasal cavity • Projection that forms anterior part of hard-palate • Conical depressions that hold roots of upper Teeth
Nasal (2)	—	• Form the bridge of the nose
Lacrimal (2)	• Lacrimal canal	• Opening for nasolacrimal duct to take tears tonasal cavity
Zygomatic (2)	—	• Form point of cheek; articulate with frontal, temporal, and maxillae
Palatine (2)	—	• Form the posterior part of hard palate
Vomer	—	• Lower part of nasal septum

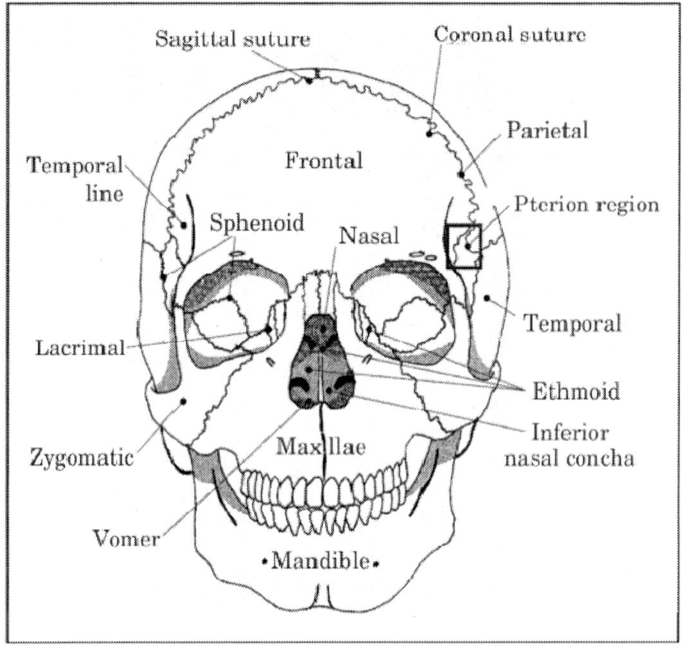

Fig. 5.1: Individual bones of cranium frontal bone

Frontal Bone

This is the bone of the forehead. It forms part of the *orbital cavities* (eye sockets) and the prominent ridges above the eyes, the *supraorbital margins.* Just above the supraorbital margins, within the bone, there are two air-filled cavities or *sinuses* lined with ciliated mucous membrane which have openings into the nasal cavity. The *coronal suture* joins the frontal and parietal bones and other fibrous joints are formed with the sphenoid, zygomatic, lacrimal, nasal and ethmoid bones. The bone originates in two parts joined in the midline by *the frontal suture.*

Parietal Bones

These bones form the sides and roof of the skull. They articulate with each other at the *sagittal suture,* with the frontal bone at the coronal suture, with the occipital bone at the *lambdoidal suture* and with the temporal bones at the *squamous sutures.* The inner surface is concave and is grooved by the brain and blood vessels.

Temporal Bones

These bones lie one on each side of the head and form immovable joints with the parietal, occipital, sphenoid and zygomatic bones. Each temporal bone has several important features. The *squamous part* is the thin fan-shaped part that articulates with the parietal bone. *The zygomatic process* articulates with the zygomatic bone to form the zygomatic arch cheekbone). The *mastoid part* contains the *mastoid process,* a thickened region behind the ear. It contains a large number of very small air sinuses which communicate with the middle ear and are lined with squamous epithelium. The *petrous portion* forms part of the base of the skull and contains the organs of hearing (the spiral organ) and balance. The temporal bone articulates with the mandible at the *temporomandibular joint,* the only movable joint of the skull. Immediately behind this articulating surface is the *external auditory meatus* (auditory canal), which passes inwards towards the petrous portion of the bone.

Occipital Bone

This bone forms the back of the head and part of the base of the skull. It has immovable joints with the parietal, temporal and sphenoid bones. Its inner surface is deeply concave and the concavity is occupied by the occipital lobes of the cerebrum and by the cerebellum. The occiput has two articular condyles that form hinge joints with the first bone of the vertebral column, the *atlas.* Between the condyles there is the *foramen magnum* (meaning Targe hole') through which the spinal cord passes into the cranial cavity.

Sphenoid Bone

This bone occupies the middle portion of the base of the skull and it articulates with the occipital, temporal, parietal and frontal bones. On the superior surface in the middle of the bone there is a little saddle-shaped depression, the *hypophyseal fossa (sella turcica)* in which the *pituitary gland* rests. The body of the bone contains some fairly large air sinuses lined by ciliated mucous membrane with openings into the nasal cavity (Fig. 5.2).

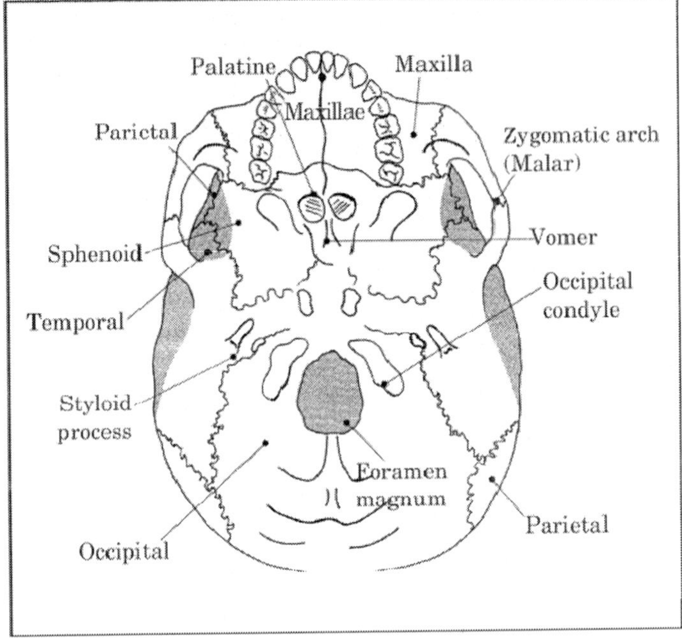

Fig. 5.2: Individual bones of cranium basal view

Ethmoid Bone

The ethmoid bone occupies the anterior part of the base of the skull and helps to form the orbital cavity, the nasal septum and the lateral walls of the nasal cavity. On each side are two projections into the nasal cavity, the *upper* and *middle conchae* or *turbinated processes.* It is a very delicate bone containing many air sinuses lined with ciliated epithelium and with openings into the nasal cavity. The horizontal flattened part, the *cribriform plate,* forms theroof of the nasal cavity and has numerous small foramina through which nerve fibres of the *olfactory nerve* (sense of smell) pass upwards from the nasal cavity to the brain. There is also a very fine *perpendicular plate* of bone that forms the upper part of the *nasal septum.*

Hyoid Bone

This is an isolated horse-shoe-shaped bone lying in the soft tissues of the neck just above the *larynx* and below the *mandible* .It does not articulate with any other bone but is attached to the styloid process of the temporal bone by ligaments. It gives attachment to the base of the tongue.

FACIAL BONES

The skeleton of the face is formed by 13 bones in addition to the frontal bone, already described.

2 Zygomatic or cheek bones
1 Maxilla (originated as 2)
2 Nasal bones
2 Lacrimal bones
1 Vomer
2 Palatine bones
2 Inferior conchae
1 Mandible (originated as 2)

Zygomatic or Cheek Bones

The zygomatic bones form the prominences of the cheeks and part of the floor and lateral walls of the orbital cavities.

Maxilla or Upper Jaw Bone

This originates as two bones but fusion takes place before birth. The maxilla forms the upper jaw, the anterior part of the roof of the mouth, the lateral walls of the nasal cavity and part of the floor of the orbital cavities. The *alveolar ridge,* or *process,* projects downwards and carries the upper teeth. On each side there is a large air sinus, the *maxillary sinus,* lined with ciliated mucous membrane and with openings into the nasal cavity.

Nasal Bones

These are two small flat bones which form the greater part of the lateral and superior surfaces of the bridge of the nose.

Lacrimal Bones

These two small bones are posterior and lateral to the nasal bones and form part of the medial walls of the orbital cavities. Each is pierced by a foramen for the passage of the *nasolacrimal duct* which carries the tears from the medial canthus of the eye to the nasal cavity.

Vomer

The vomer is a thin flat bone which extends upwards from the middle of the hard palate to form the main part of the nasal septum. Superiorly it articulates with the perpendicular plate of the ethmoid bone.

Palatine Bones

These are two L-shaped bones. The horizontal parts unite to form the posterior part of the hard palate and the perpendicular parts project upwards to form part of the lateral walls of the nasal cavity. At their upper extremities they form part of the orbital cavities.

Inferior Conchae

Each concha is a scroll-shaped bone which forms part of the lateral wall of the nasal cavity and projects into it below the middle concha. The superior and middle conchae are parts of the ethmoid bone.

Mandible

This is the only movable bone of the skull. It originates as two parts which unite at the midline. Each half consists of two main parts: a *curved body* with the *alveolar ridge* containing the lower teeth and a *ramus* which projects upwards almost at right angles to the posterior end of the body.

At the upper end the ramus divides into the *condilar process* which articulates with the temporal bone to form the *temporomandibular* joint and the *coronoid process* that gives attachment to muscles and ligaments. The point where the ramus joins the body is the *angle* of the jaw.

BONES OF THORACIC CAGE

The skeleton framework of the thorax is formed by the thoracic vertebrae in the back side and sternum costal cartilages and ribs in front.

The bones of the thorax or thoracic cage are: (Fig. 5.3)

1 Sternum

12 Pairs of ribs

12 Thoracic vertebrae.

Ribs and Costal Cartilages

There are 12 pairs of ribs, which are numbered 1 through 12, starting with the most superior rib. All of the ribs articulate posteriorly with the thoracic vertebrae. *Costal cartilages* attach many of the ribs anteriorly to the sternum. Movement of the ribs relative to the vertebrae and the flexibility of the costal cartilages allow the thoracic cage to change shape during breathing. The ribs are classified by their anterior attachments as true or false ribs.

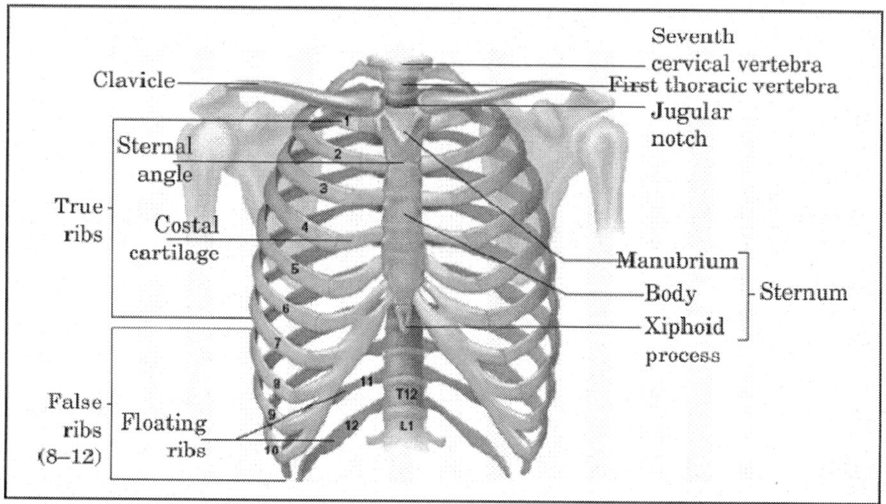

Fig. 5.3: Thoracic cage

***The true ribs*:** The true ribs attach directly through their costal cartilages to the sternum. The superior seven pairs of ribs are true ribs.

***The false ribs*:** The false ribs do not attach to the sternum. The inferior five pairs of ribs are false ribs. On each side, the three superior false ribs are joined by a common cartilage to the costal cartilage of the seventh true rib, which in turn is attached to the sternum.

***Floating ribs*:** The two inferior pairs of false ribs are also called *floating* **ribs** because they do not attach to the sternum.

The Typical Rib

Most ribs have two points of articulation with the thoracic vertebrae (Fig. 5.4).

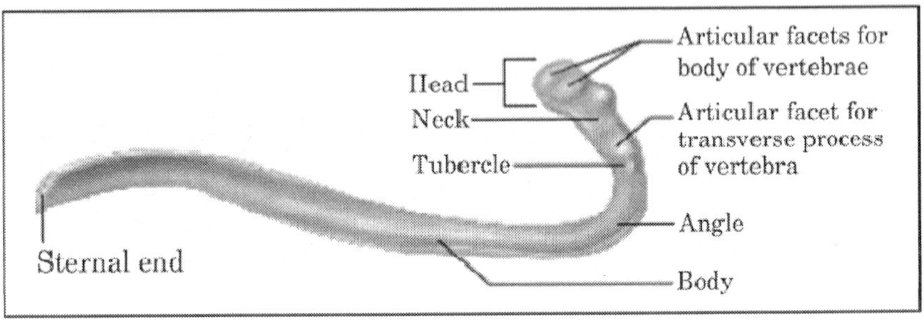

Fig. 5.4: The typical rib

First, the *head* articulates with the bodies of two adjacent vertebrae and the intervertebral disk between them. The head of each rib articulates with the inferior articular facet of the superior vertebra and the superior articular facet of the inferior vertebra. Second, the *tubercle* articulates with the transverse process of the inferior vertebra. The *neck* is between the head and tubercle, and the *body,* or shaft, is the main part of the rib. The *angle* of the rib is located just lateral to the tubercle and is the point of greatest curvature.

Sternum

The *sternum*, or breastbone, has three parts: the *manubrium* (handle), the *body*, and the *xiphoid* (sword) *process*. The sternum resembles a sword, with the manubrium forming the handle, the body forming the blade, and the xiphoid process forming the tip. At the superior end of the sternum, a depression, called the *jugular notch*, is located between the ends of the clavicles where they articulate with the manubrium of the sternum. The jugular notch can easily be found at the base of the neck. A slight ridge, called the *sternal angle*, can be felt at the junction of the manubrium and the body of the sternum.

Experiment No. 6

AIM: To Study the Bones of Vertebral Column

Key words: Vertebral column, Typical vertebra,

The vertebral (*verto,* to turn) column, or backbone, is the central axis of the skeleton, extending from the base of the skull to slightly past the end of the pelvis. The vertebral column performs five major functions: (1) It supports the weight of the head and trunk, (2) It protects the spinal cord, (3) It allows spinal nerves to exit the spinal cord, (4) It provides a site for muscle attachment, and (5) It permits movement of the head and trunk.

Different Regions of Vertebral Column:

The vertebral column usually consists of 26 individual bones, grouped into five regions

- 7 Cervical (neck) vertebrae,
- 12 Thoracic (chest) vertebrae,
- 5 Lumbar (loin) vertebrae,
- 1 Sacral (sacred) bone,
- 1 Coccygeal (shaped like a cuckoo's bill) bone make up the vertebral 'column.

Curves of the Vertebral Column

When viewed from the side the vertebral column presents four curves, two *primary* and two *secondary*. The fetus in the uterus lies curled up so that the head and the knees are more or less touching. This position shows the *primary curvature*. The secondary *cervical curve* develops when the child can hold up his head (after about 3 months) and the secondary *lumbar curve* develops when he stands upright (after 12 to 15 months). The thoracic and sacral primary curves are retained.

Functions of the Vertebral Column

- These include the following.
- Collectively the vertebral foramina form the vertebral canal which provides a strong bony protection for the delicate spinal cord lying within it.
- The pedicles of adjacent vertebrae form intervertebral foramina, one on each side, providing access to the spinal cord for spinal nerves, blood vessels and lymph vessels
- The numerous individual bones enable a certain amount of movement.
- It supports the skull.
- The intervertebral discs act as shock absorbers, protecting the brain.
- It forms the axis of the trunk, giving attachment to the ribs, shoulder girdle and upper limbs, and the pelvic girdle and lower limbs.

Cervical Vertebrae

The *cervical vertebrae* all have a *transverse foramen* in each transverse process through which the vertebral arteries extend toward the head.

Atlas: The first cervical vertebra is called the *Atlas* (Fig. 6.1) because it holds up the head, just as Atlas in classical mythology held up the world. The atlas has no body, but it has large superior articular facets where it articulates with the occipital condyles on the base of the skull. This joint allows the head to move in a “yes” motion or to tilt from side to side.

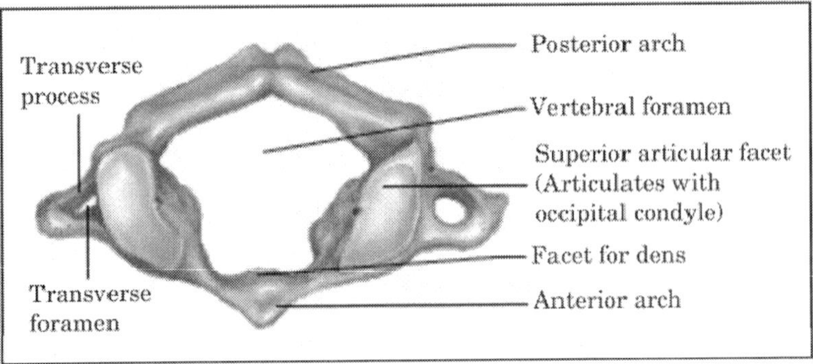

Fig. 6.1: Atlas

Axis: The second cervical vertebra is called the *axis* (Fig. 6.2) because it has a projection around which the atlas rotates to produce a "no" motion of the head. The projection is called the *dens* (denz, toothshaped) or *odontoid* (tooth-shaped), *process*. The atlas does not have a spinous process.

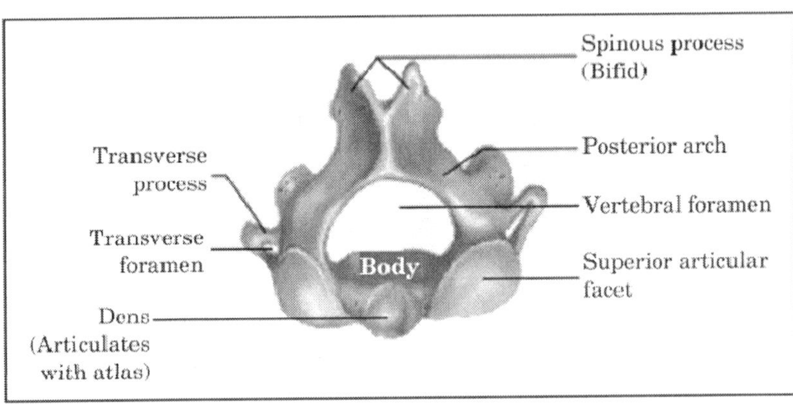

Fig. 6.2: Axis

The spinous process of most cervical vertebrae end in two parts and are called *bifid* (split) *spinous processes* (Fig. 6.3). The spinous process of the seventh cervical vertebra is not bifid; it is often quite pronounced and often can be seen and felt as a lump between the shoulders called the *vertebra prominens*. Although the vertebra prominens usually marks the division between the cervical and thoracic vertebrae, sometimes it is part of the sixth cervical vertebra or the first thoracic vertebra.

Table 6.1: General Structure of a Vertebra

Feature	***Description***
Body	Disk-shaped; usually the largest part. with flat surfaces directed superiorly and inferiorly; forms the anterior wall of the vertebral foramen;intervertebral disks are located between the bodies
Vertebral foramen	Hole in each vertebra through which the spinal cord passes; adjacent vertebral foramina form the vertebral canal
Vertebral arch	Forms the lateral and posterior walls of the vertebral foramen; possesses several processes and articular surfaces
Pedicle	Foot of the arch with one on each side; forms the lateral walls of the vertebral foramen
Lamina	Posterior part of the arch; forms the posterior wall of the vertebral foramen
Transverse process	Process projecting laterally from the junction of the lamina and pedicle; a site of muscle attachment
Spinous process	Process projecting posteriorly at the point where the two laminae join; a site of muscle attachment; strengthens the vertebral column and allows for movement
Articular processes	Superior and inferior projections containing articular facets where vertebrae articulate with each other; strengthen the vertebral column and allow for movement
Intervertebral notches	Form intervertebral foramina between two adjacent vertebrae through which spinal nerves exit the vertebral canal

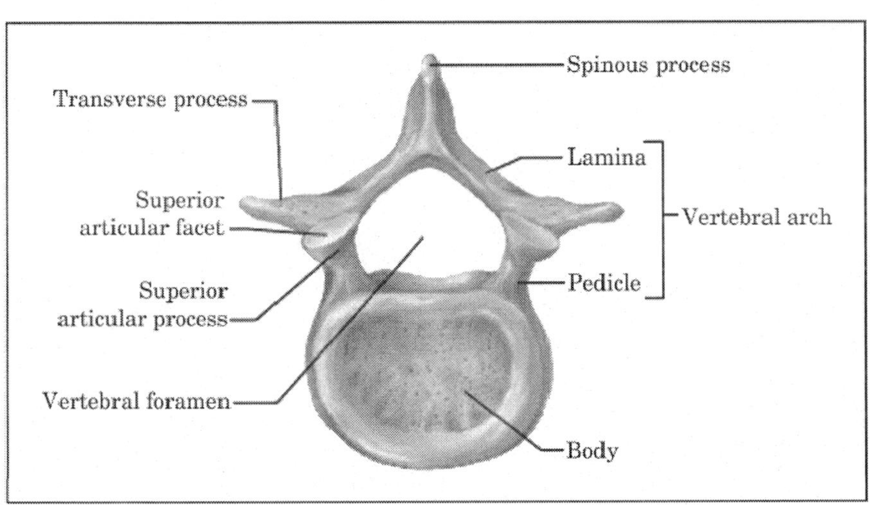

***Thoracic vertebrae*:** The *thoracic vertebrae* (Fig. 6.4) have attachment sites for the ribs. The first 10 thoracic vertebrae have articular facets on their transverse processes, where they articulate with the tubercles of the ribs. Additional articular facets are on

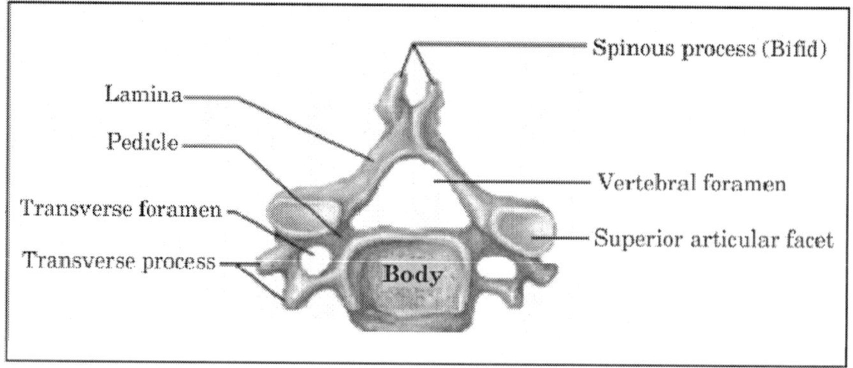

Fig. 6.3: Cervical vertebrae

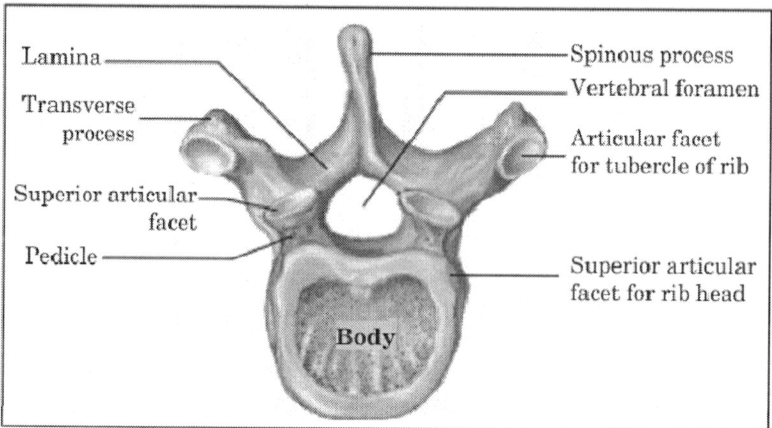

Fig. 6.4: Thoracic vertebrae

the superior and articular inferior margins of the body where the heads of the ribs articulate. Thoracic vertebrae have long, thin spinous processes, which are directed inferiorly.

***Lumbar Vertebrae*:** The *lumbar vertebrae* (Fig. 6.5) have large, thick bodies and heavy, rectangular transverse and spinous processes. The superior articular facets face medially, and the inferior articular facets face laterally. When the superior articular surface of one lumbar vertebra joins the inferior articulating surface of another lumbar vertebra, the arrangement tends to "lock" adjacent lumbar vertebrae together, giving the lumbar part of the vertebral column more stability and limiting rotation of the lumbar vertebrae. The articular facets in other regions of the vertebral column have a more “open” position, allowing for more movement but less stability.

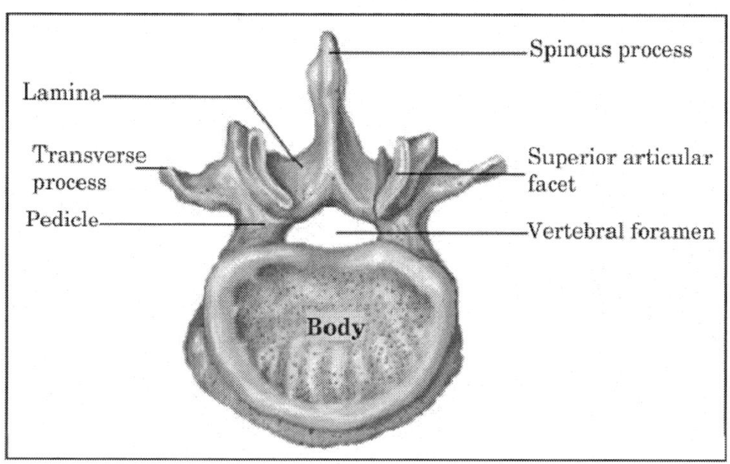

Fig. 6.5: Lumbar vertebrae

The five *sacral vertebrae* are fused into a single bone called the *sacrum*. Although the margins of the sacral bodies unite after the twentieth year, the interior of the sacrum is not ossified until midlife. The transverse processes fuse to form the lateral parts of the sacrum. The superior lateral part of the sacrum forms wing-shaped areas called the *alae* (wings). Much of the lateral surfaces of the sacrum are ear shaped *auricular surfaces*, which join the sacrum to the pelvic bones. The spinous processes of the first four sacral vertebrae partially fuse to form projections, called the *median sacral crest*. The spinous process of the fifth sacral vertebra does not form, thereby leaving a *sacral hiatus*, or gap, which exposes the sacral canal. The vertebral canal within the sacrum is called the sacral canal. The sacral hiatus is used to gain entry into the sacral canal to administer anesthetic injections—for example, just before childbirth. The anterior edge of the body of the first sacral vertebra bulges to form the sacral promontory, a landmark that separates the abdominal cavity from the pelvic cavity. Th e sacral promontory can be felt during a vaginal examination, and it is used as a reference point during measurement to determine if the pelvic openings are large enough to allow for normal vaginal delivery of a baby.

The coccyx (kok2 siks, shaped like a cuckoo's bill), or tailbone, usually consists of four more or less fused vertebrae. The vertebrae of the coccyx do not have the typical structure of most other vertebrae. They consist of extremely reduced vertebral bodies, without the foramina or processes, usually fused into a single bone.

Table 6.2: Comparison of vertebral regions

Feature	*Cervical*	*Thoracic*	*Lumbar*
Body	Absent in C1, small in others	Medium-sized with articular facets for ribs	Large
Transverse process	Transverse foramen	Articular facets for ribs, except T11 and T12	Square
Spinous process	Absent in C1, bifid in others, except C7	Long, angled inferiorly	Square
Articular facets	Face superior/inferior	Face obliquely	Face medial/ lateral

Experiment No. 7

AIM: To Study the Bones of Pectoral Girdle and Upper Limb Pectoral Girdle

***Key words*:** Humerus , Radius, Ulna , Carpal bones, Metacarpal bones, Phalanges

PECTORAL GIRDLE

The *pectoral girdle,* or *shoulder girdle*, consists of two *scapulae*, or shoulder blades, and two clavicles (klav2 i-klz, key), or collarbones. Each Humerus (arm bone) attaches to a scapula, which is connected by a clavicle to the sternum. The scapula is a flat, triangular bone that can easily be seen and felt in a living person. The *glenoid* (glen2 oyd) *cavity* is a depression where the humerus connects to the scapula. The scapula has three fossae where muscles extending to the arm are attached. The *scapular spine*, which runs across the posterior surface of the scapula, separates two of these fossae. The *supraspinous fossa* is superior to the spine and the *infraspinous fossa* is inferior to it. The *subscapular fossa* is on the anterior surface of the scapula. The *acromion* (*akron,* tip + *omos,* shoulder) is an extension of the spine forming the point of the shoulder. The acromion forms a protective cover for the shoulder joint and is the attachment site for the clavicle and some of the shoulder muscles. The *coracoid* (crow's beak) *process* curves below the clavicle and provides attachment for arm and chest muscles.

UPPER LIMB

Each upper limb consists of the following bones:

1 Humerus

1 Radius
1 Ulna
8 Carpal bones
5 Metacarpal bones
14 Phalanges

BONES OF PECTORAL GIRDLE

Clavicle

The clavicle is a long bone with a slight sigmoid (S-shaped) curve and is easily seen and felt in the living human. The *acromial (lateral) end* of the clavicle articulates with the acromion of the scapula, and the *sternal (medial) end* articulates with the manubrium of the sternum. The pectoral girdle's only attachment to the axial skeleton is at the sternum. Mobility of the upper limb is enhanced by movement of the scapula, which is possible because the clavicle can move relative to the sternum. For example, feel the movement of the clavicle when shrugging the shoulders.

Scapula or Shoulder Blade

The scapula is a flat triangular-shaped bone, lying on the posterior chest wall superficial to the ribs and separated from them by muscles. At the lateral angle there is a shallow articular surface, the *glenoid cavity* which, with the *head of the humerus,* forms the *shoulder joint.*

On the posterior surface there is a *spinous process* that projects beyond the lateral angle of the bone that overhangs the shoulder joint, called the *acromion process.* It articulates with the clavicle at the *acromiodavicular joint.* The *coracoid process,* a projection from the upper border of the bone, gives attachment to muscles that move the shoulder joint. (Fig. 7.1)

BONES OF UPPER LIMB

Humerus

The humeral *head* articulates with the glenoid cavity of the scapula. The *anatomical neck*, around the head of the humerus, is where

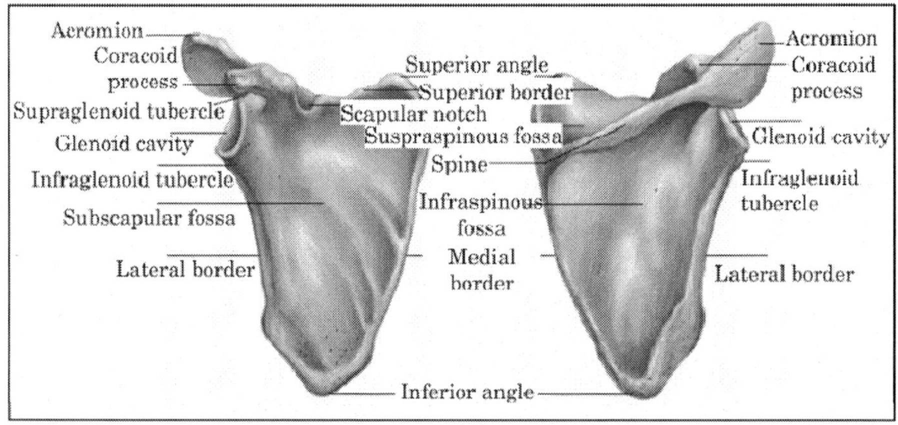

Fig. 7.1: Scapula or Shoulder blade

connective tissue holding the shoulder joint together attaches. The *surgical neck* is so named because it is a common fracture site that often requires surgical repair. If it becomes necessary to remove the humeral head because of disease or injury, it is removed down to the surgical neck. The *greater tubercle* and the *lesser tubercle* are sites of muscle attachment. The *intertubercular groove*, or *bicipital groove*, between the tubercles contains one tendon of the biceps brachii muscle. The *deltoid tuberosity* is located on the lateral surface of the humerus a little more than a third of the way along its length and is the attachment site for the deltoid muscle. Condyles on the distal end of the humerus articulate with the two forearm bones. The *capitulum* (head-shaped) is very rounded and articulates with the radius. The *trochlea* (spool) somewhat resembles a spool or pulley and articulates with the ulna. Proximal to the capitulum and the trochlea are the *medial* and *lateral epicondyles*, which are points of muscle attachment for the muscles of the forearm. They can be found as bony protuberances proximal to the elbow (Fig. 7.2).

Ulna and Radius

The *ulna* is on the medial (little finger) side of the forearm, whereas the *radius* is on the lateral (thumb) side of the forearm. The proximal end of the ulna has a C-shaped articular surface called

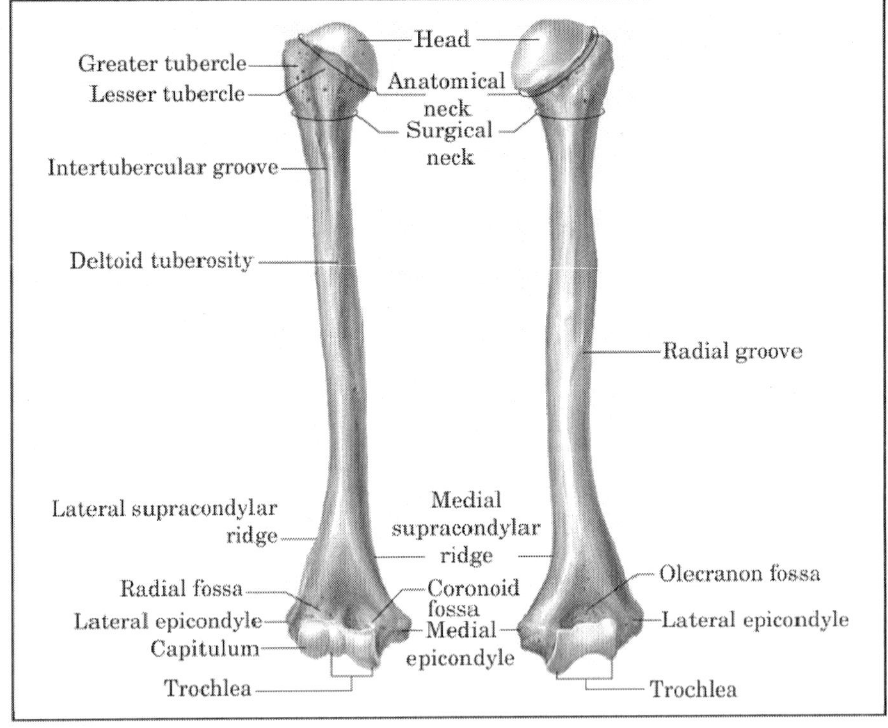

Fig. 7.2: Humerus

the *trochlear notch*, or *semilunar notch that* fits over the trochlea of the humerus, forming most of the elbow joint. The trochlear notch is bounded by two processes. The *olecranon* (the point of the elbow) is the posterior process forming the tip of the elbow. It can easily be felt and is commonly referred to as "the elbow." Posterior arm muscles attach to the olecranon. The smaller, anterior process is the *coronoid* (crow's beak) *process*. The proximal end of the radius is the *head*. It is concave and articulates with the capitulum of the humerus. Movements of the radial head relative to the capitulum and of the trochlear notch relative to the trochlea allow the elbow to bend and straighten. The lateral surfaces of the radial head form a smooth cylinder where the radius rotates against the *radial notch* of the ulna. As the forearm supinates and pronates the proximal end of the ulna stays in place and the radius rotates. Just distal to the elbow joint, the *radial tuberosity* and the *ulnar tuberosity* are attachment sites for arm muscles. The distal end of the ulna has a small *head*, which articulates with both the radius and the carpal (wrist) bones. The head can be seen as a prominent lump on the posterior, medial (ulnar) side of the distal forearm. The distal end of the radius, which articulates with the ulna and the carpal bones, is somewhat broadened. The ulna and radius have small *styloid* (shaped like a stylus or writing instrument) *processes* to which ligaments of the wrist are attached (Fig 7.3).

Carpal or Wrist Bones

The wrist is a relatively short region between the forearm and hand; it is composed of eight *carpal bones* arranged into two rows of four each. The proximal row of carpal bones, lateral to medial,

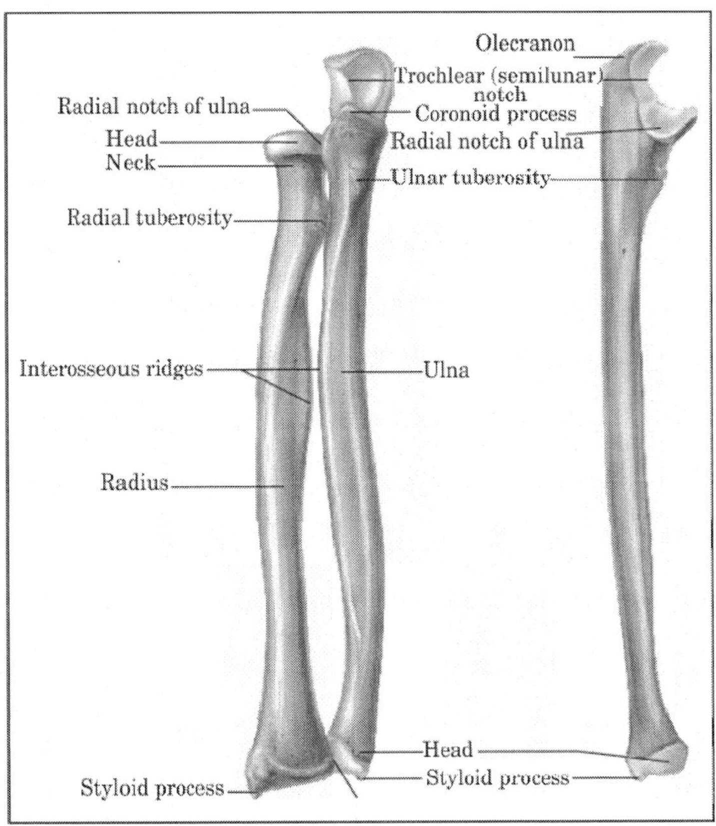

Fig. 7.3: Radius and Ulna

includes the *scaphoid* (boat-shaped), *lunate* (moon-shaped), *triquetrum* (three-cornered), and *pisiform* (pea-shaped). The distal row of carpal bones, from medial to lateral, includes the *hamate* (hook), *capitate* (head), *trapezoid* (a four-sided geometric form with two parallel sides), and *trapezium* (a four-sided geometric form with no two sides parallel). A number of mnemonics have been developed to help students remember the carpal bones. The following mnemonic allows students to remember them in order from lateral to medial for the proximal row (top) and from medial to lateral (by the thumb) for the distal row: So Long Top Part, Here Comes The Thumb—that is Scaphoid, Lunate, Triquetrum, Pisiform, Hamate, Capitate, Trapezoid, and Trapezium. (Fig. 7.4).

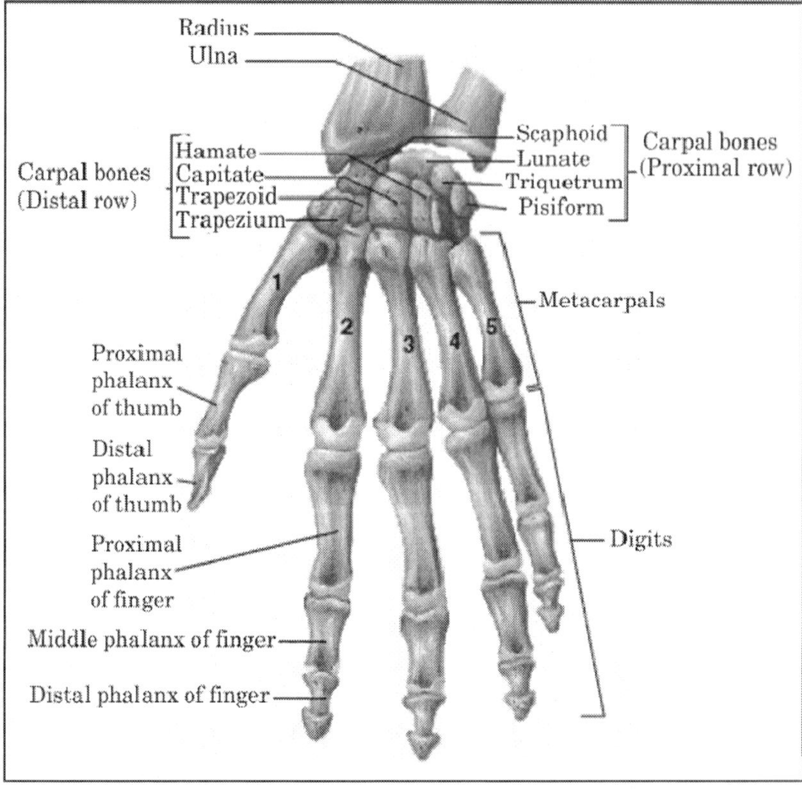

Fig. 7.4: Carpals and Metacarpal

Metacarpal

Five *metacarpal* (after the carpals) *bones* are attached to the carpal bones and constitute the bony framework of the hand. They are numbered 1 through 5, starting with the most lateral metacarpal, at the base of the thumb. The distal ends of the metacarpal bones help form the knuckles of the hand.

Phalanges

The five *digits* of each hand include one thumb and four fingers. The digits are also numbered 1 through 5, starting from the thumb. Each digit consists of small long bones called *phalanges* (sing. *phalanx,* a line or wedge of soldiers holding their spears, tips outward, in front of them). The thumb has two phalanges, called proximal and distal. Each finger has three phalanges designated proximal, middle, and distal. One or two *sesamoid* (resembling a sesame seed) *bones* often form near the junction between the proximal phalanx and the metacarpal of the thumb. Sesamoid bones are small bones located within some tendons, increasing their mechanical advantage where they cross joints.

Experiment No. 8

AIM: To Study the Bones of Pelvic Girdle and Lower Limb

***Key words*:** Pelvic bones, Male and female pelvis, Femur, Tibia fibula, Patella, Tarsals, Metatarsals, Phalanges

The pelvic girdle is the place of attachment for the lower limbs, it supports the weight of the body, and it protects internal organs. The right and left *coxal bones*, or coxae, or hipbones, join each other anteriorly and the *sacrum* posteriorly to form a ring of bone called the *pelvic girdle* (Fig. 8.1a). The *pelvis* (basin) includes the pelvic girdle and the coccyx. Because the pelvic girdle is a complete bony ring, it provides more stable support but less mobility than the incomplete ring of the pectoral girdle. In addition, the pelvis in a woman protects a developing fetus and forms a passageway through which the fetus passes during delivery. Each coxal bone is formed by three bones fused to one another to form a single bone. The *ilium* (groin) is the superior, the *ischium* (hip) is inferior and posterior, and the *pubis* (genital hair) is inferior and anterior (Fig. 8.1b).

The coxal bones join anteriorly at the *symphysis* (a coming together) *pubis*, or *pubic symphysis*. Posteriorly, each coxal bone joins the sacrum at the *sacroiliac joint*.

A fossa called the *acetabulum* (a shallow vinegar cup—a common household item in ancient times) is located on the lateral surface of each coxal bone. In a child, the joints between the ilium, ischium, and pubis can be seen. The bones fuse together in some locations by the seventh or eighth year. Complete fusion within the acetabulum occurs between the sixteenth and eighteenth years.

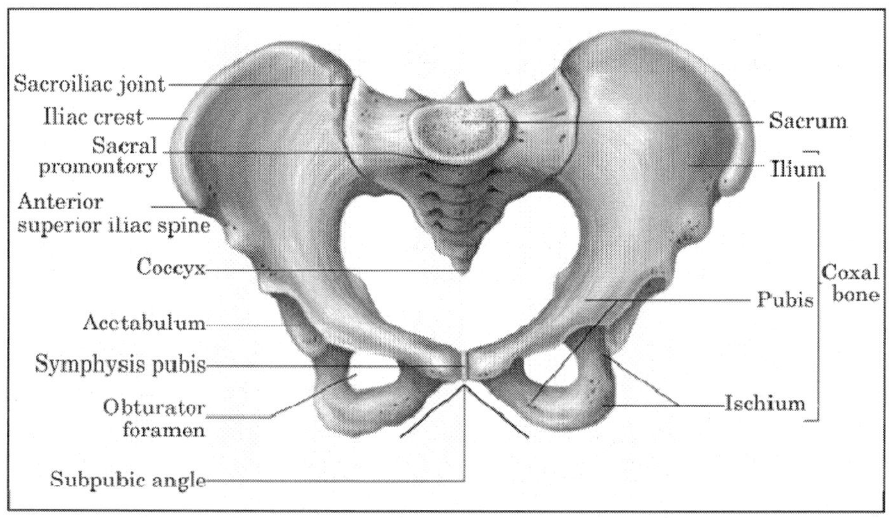

Fig. 8.1a: Pelvis

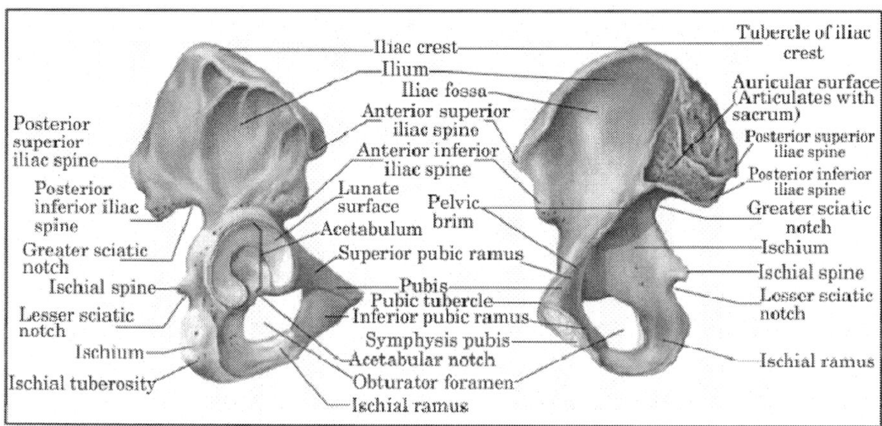

Fig. 8.1b: Coxal or Hip Bone

The acetabulum is the point of articulation of the lower limb with the pelvic girdle. The articular, *lunate surface* of the acetabulum is crescent-shaped and occupies only the superior and lateral aspects of the fossa. Inferior to the acetabulum is the large *obturator* (to occlude or close up) *foramen.*

In life, the obturator foramen is almost completely closed off by a connective tissue membrane, which separates the pelvic cavity from more superficial structures. Despite its large size, only a few small blood vessels and nerves pass through the obturator foramen. The superior portion of the ilium is called the *iliac crest*. The crest ends anteriorly as the *anterior superior iliac spine* and posteriorly as the *posterior superior iliac spine*. The crest and anterior spine can be felt and even seen in thin individuals. The anterior superior iliac spine is an important anatomical landmark used, for example, to find the correct location for giving gluteal injections into the hip. A dimple overlies the posterior superior iliac spine just superior to the buttocks. Inferior to the anterior superior iliac spine is the *anterior inferior iliac spine*. The anterior iliac spines are attachment sites for anterior thigh muscles. Inferior to the superior posterior iliac spine are the *posterior inferior iliac spine, ischial spine*, and ischial tuberosity. The posterior iliac spines and ischial tuberosity are attachment sites for ligaments anchoring the coxal bone to the sacrum. The *auricular surface* of the ilium joins the auricular surface of the sacrum to form the sacroiliac joint. Th e ischial tuberosity is also an attachment site for posterior thigh muscles, and it is the part of the coxal bone on which a person sits. The *greater sciatic notch* is superior to the ischial spine and the *lesser sciatic notch* is inferior to it. Nerves and blood vessels pass through the sciatic notches. The pelvis is divided into the *false pelvis* and the *true pelvis* by an imaginary plane passing from the sacral promontory to the pubic crest. The *pelvic brim* is the bony boundary of this plane. The false pelvis, which is the expanded part of the pelvis superior to the pelvic brim, is also the inferior part of the abdominal cavity. The true pelvis is inferior to the pelvic brim and is completely surrounded by bone. The *pelvic inlet* is the superior opening of the true pelvis formed by the pelvic brim. The *pelvic outlet* is the inferior opening of the true pelvis bordered by the inferior margin of the pubis, the ischial spines, the ischial tuberosities, and the coccyx. The *pelvic cavity* is the space between the pelvic inlet and the pelvic diaphragm.

Comparison of the Male and Female Pelvis

The male pelvis (Fig. 8.2) usually is more massive than the female pelvis (Fig. 8.3) as a result of the greater weight and size of the male, but the female pelvis is broader and has a larger, more rounded pelvic inlet and outlet consistent with the need to allow

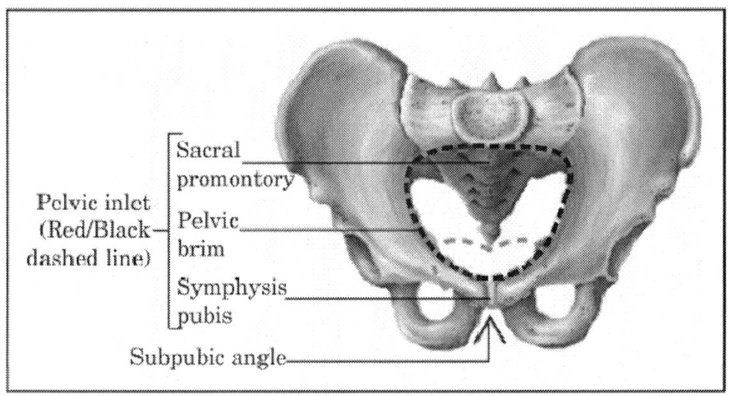

Fig. 8.2: Male Pelvis

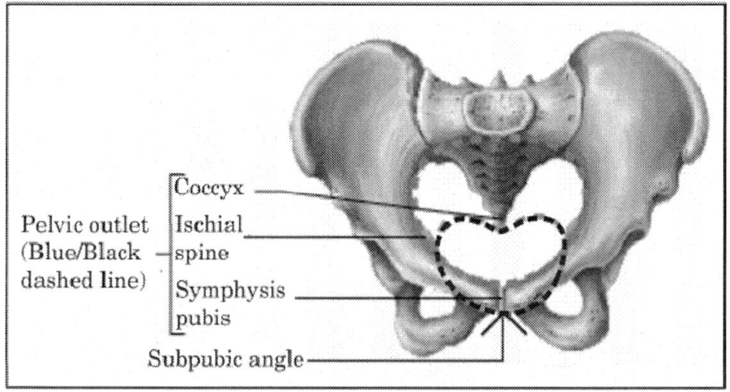

Fig. 8.3: Female Pelvis

a fetus to pass through these openings in the female pelvis during delivery (Table 8.1). If the pelvic outlet is too small for normal delivery, it can be accomplished by cesarean section, which is the surgical removal of the fetus through the abdominal wall.

LOWER LIMB

The bones of the lower limb are:

- 1 Femur • 7 Tarsal bones
- 1 Tibia • 5 Metatarsal bones
- 1 Fibula • 14 Phalanges.
- 1 Patella

Table 8.1: Comparison of the male and female Pelvis

Area	*Description for Female*	*Description for Male*
General	Light and thin	Heavy and thick
False pelvis	Shallow	Deep
Pelvic brim	Larger and more oval	Smaller and heart shaped
Acetabulum	Small and faces anteriorly	Larger and faces laterally
Obturator foramen	Oval	Round
Pubic arch	90 degrees or more in females	Less than 90 degrees in males
Iliac crest	Less curved	More curved
Ilium	Less verticle	More verticle
Obturator foramen	Triangular	Oval
Greater sciatic notch	Wide	Narrow
Coccyx	More moveable and more curved anteriorly	Less moveable and less curved anteriorly
Sacrum	Shorter wide and more curved anteriorly	Longer narrow and less curved anteriorly

Femur or Thigh Bone

The femur is the longest and strongest bone of the body (Fig. 8.4). The head is almost spherical and fits into the *acetabulum* of the hip bone to form the *hip joint*. In the centre of the head there is a small depression for the attachment of the *ligament of the head of the femur*. This extends from the acetabulum to the femur and contains a blood vessel that supplies blood to an area of the head of the bone. The neck extends outwards and slightly downwards from the head to the shaft and most of it is within the capsule of the hip joint. The posterior surface of the lower third forms a flat triangular area called the *popliteal surface*. The distal extremity has two articular *condyles* which, with the tibia and patella, form the knee joint.

Tibia or Shin Bone

The tibia is the medial of the two bones of the lower leg (Fig. 8.5). The proximal extremity is broad and flat and presents two *condoles* for articulation with the femur at the *knee joint*. The head of the fibula articulates with the inferior aspect of the lateral condyle, forming the *proximal tibiofibular* joint. The distal extremity of the

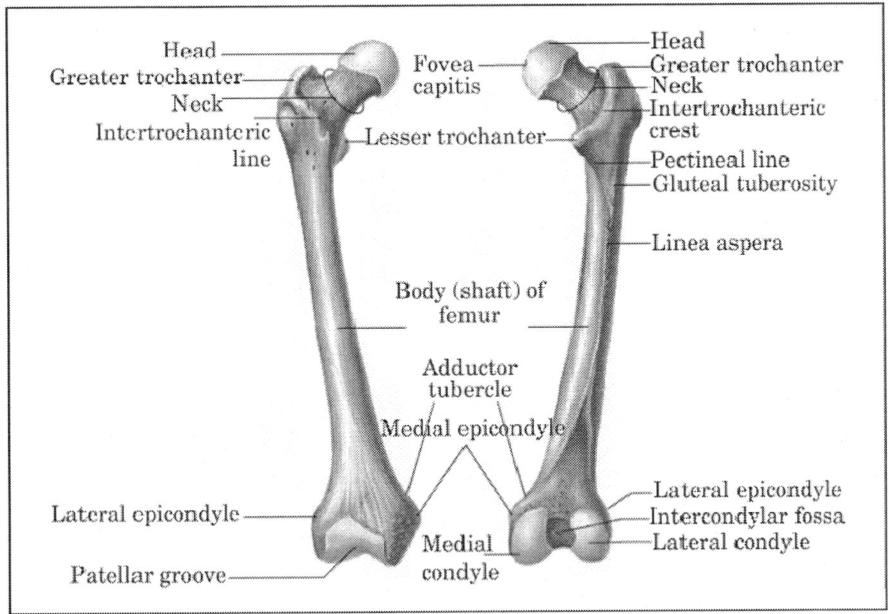

Fig. 8.4: Femur

tibia forms the *ankle joint* with the *talus* and the fibula. The *medial malleolus* is a downward projection of bone medial to the ankle joint.

Fibula

The fibula is the long slender lateral bone in the leg (Fig. 8.5). The head or upper extremity articulates with the lateral condyle of the tibia forming the proximal tibiofibular joint and the lower extremity articulates with the tibia then projects beyond it to form the *lateral malleolus.*

Patella or Knee Cap

This is a roughly triangular-shaped *sesamoid* bone associated with the knee joint. Its posterior surface articulates with the patellar surface of the femur in the knee joint and its anterior surface is in the *patellar tendon, i.e.* the tendon of the quadriceps femoris muscle.

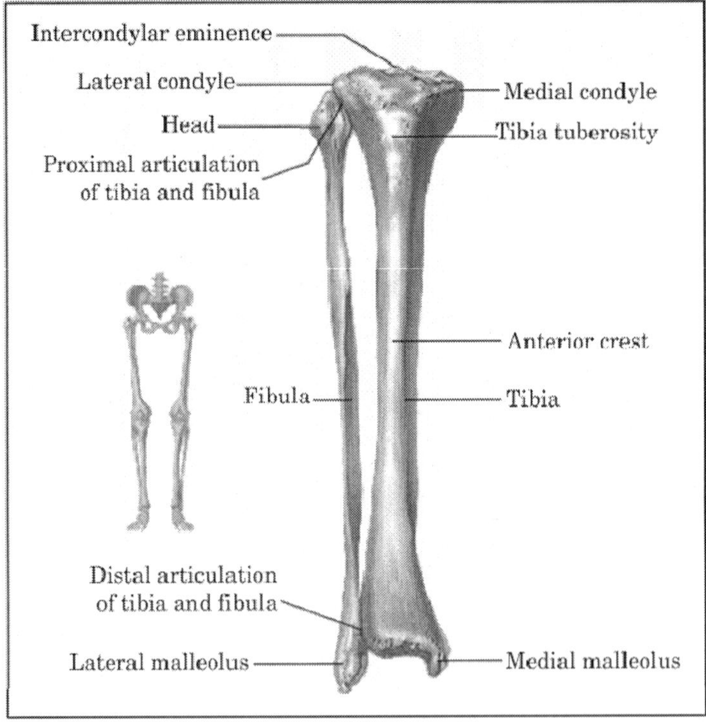

Fig. 8.5: Tibia and Fibula

Tarsal or Ankle Bones

There are seven tarsal bones which form the posterior part of the foot (Fig. 8.6). They are:

- 1 Talus • 3 Cuneiform
- 1 Calcaneus • 1 Cuboid.
- 1 Navicular

The *talus* articulates with the tibia and fibula at the ankle joint. The *calcaneus* forms the heel of the foot. The other bones articulate with each other and with the metatarsal bones.

Metatarsal Bones of the Foot

These are five bones, numbered from within outwards, which form the greater part of the dorsum of the foot. At their proximal ends

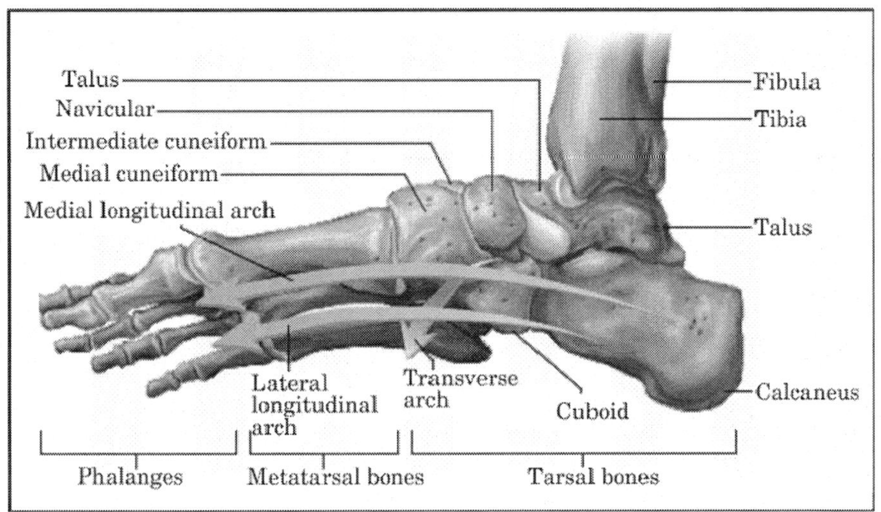

Fig. 8.6: Bones of foot

they articulate with the tarsal bones and at their distal ends, with the phalanges. The enlarged distal head of the 1st metatarsal bone forms the 'ball' of the foot.

Phalanges of the Toes

There are 14 phalanges arranged in a similar manner to those in the fingers, *i.e.* two in the great toe (the *halux)* and three in each of the other toes.

Arches of the Foot

The arrangement of the bones of the foot is such that it is not a rigid structure. This point is well illustrated by comparing a normal foot with a 'flat' foot. The bones have a bridge-like arrangement and are supported by muscles and ligaments so that four arches are formed, a *medial* and *lateral longitudinal arch* and two *transverse arches.*

Medial longitudinal arch: This is the highest of the arches and is formed by the calcaneus, talus, navicular, three cuneiform and first three metatarsal bones. Only the calcaneus and the distal end of the metatarsal bones should touch the ground.

Lateral longitudinal arch: The lateral arch is much less marked than its medial counterpart. The bony components are the calcaneus, cuboid and the two lateral metatarsal bones. Again only the calcaneus and metatarsal bones should touch the ground.

Transverse arches: These run across the foot and can be more easily seen by examining the skeleton than the live model. They are most marked at the level of the three cuneiform and cuboid bones.

Experiment No. 9

Aim: To Study the Introduction of Hematology

***Key words*:** Blood, Functions and Properties, Composition, Collection of Blood Sample: Venous and Capillary Blood

HEMATOLOGY

Hematology (Greek Hema = Blood; logy = Study of). Hematology is the branch of medical science that deals with the study of blood. *Blood*, along with the *cardiovascular system* constitutes the *Circulatory system* and performs the following functions:

1. ***Transport*:** Blood provides a pickup and delivery system for the transport of gases, nutrients, hormones, waste products, etc. over a route of some 1,12,000 km of blood vessels, with 60–70 trillion customers (cells).
2. ***Regulation*:** It regulates the body temperature by transporting heat from the tissues (mainly liver and muscles) to the skin from where it can be lost. Its buffers regulate pH of the body fluids, while its osmotic pressure regulates water content of cells through the actions of its dissolved proteins and ions.
3. ***Protection*:** The blood protects the body against diseases caused by harmful organisms by transporting leukocytes and antibodies against more than a million foreign invaders. It also protects the body against loss of blood after injury by the process of blood clotting.

Physical Properties of Blood

The blood is denser and more viscous than water, slightly alkaline, sticky to touch, and salty in taste. It clots on standing, leaving behind serum. The normal total circulating blood volume amounts to 8% of the body weight, *i.e.* 5–6 litres in an average adult male weighing 70 kg, and 4–5 litres in a female. The interplay of various hormones that control salt and water excretion in the urine keep the blood volume remarkably constant.

Its color varies from bright red in the arteries and when exposed to the air, to various tints from dark purple to red in the veins. The color of the blood is due to the coloring constituent of the red corpuscles, *hæmoglobin*, which is brighter or darker as it contains more or less oxygen.

Components of Blood

Blood plasma is a straw-coloured (yellowish) liquid, which makes up about 55% of total blood volume after the sedimentation of formed elements in a blood sample. It contains approx. 91.5% water and 8.5% solutes, most of which are proteins like albumins, globulins or fibrinogen. Antibodies or immunoglobulins belong to the group of globulins, and play important role during certain immune responses. Besides proteins, other solutes like electrolytes, nutrients, waste products, regulatory substances and gases are also present.

Formed elements include three principal components: *red blood cells* (RBCs or erythrocytes; 4.8-5.4 million/μl blood), *white blood cells* (WBCs or leukocytes; 500-1.000/μl blood) and *platelets* (thrombocytes; 150.000-400.000/μl blood). While RBCs and WBCs are whole cells, platelets are only cell fragments.

The percentage of total blood volume occupied by formed elements, mostly RBCs is called the *hematocrit*, with a normal range of 38-46% or 40-54% in case of healthy adult females or males, respectively. RBCs are biconcave discs (doughnut shape) with a diameter of 7-8 μm. In their mature form, they lack a nucleus. They contain large amount of hemoglobin molecules, which play an important role in the transport of respiratory gases. RBCs live around 120 days within the circulation. The ruptured cells are removed and destroyed by macrophages in the spleen and liver.

WBCs have nuclei and all cellular organelles and are classified as either granular or aglanular, depending on whether they contain cytoplasmic granules that can be visualised by staining. *Granular leukocytes* include neutrophils, eosinophils and basophils, depending on the type of dyes staining their granules. Their nuclei have lobes, connected by thin strands of nuclear material. *Neutrophils* (60-70% of WBCs) are active in phagocytosis, thus, they can ingest bacteria and dispose of dead cellular matter. Besides engulfing bacteria, these cells are able to release several chemicals that help to destroy pathogenic intruders. In case of an inflammation, neutrophils are able to leave the blood stream to fight injury or infection. *Eosinophils* (2-4% of WBCs) are also able to leave the capillaries and enter tissue fluid. They can phagocytize antigen-antibody complexes and are effective against certain parasites. They can also release substances involved in inflammation during allergic reactions. *Basophils* (0.5-1% of WBCs) can also leave capillaries at the sites of inflammations. They release granules that contain heparin, histamin and serotonin, which intensify inflammatory reactions and are involved in hypersensitivity (allergic) conditions.

Agranular leukocytes include lymphocytes and monocytes. *Lymphocytes* (20-25% of WBCs) have a round nucleus which almost completely fills out the cytoplasm. Their average size is 6-14 µm. They can continuously circulate between blood, tissues and lymphatic fluid and under normal conditions, only their 2% is present in the bloodstream at any given time. There are 3 main types of them. *T cells* attack viruses, fungi, some bacteria, transplanted or cancerous cells and are responsible for transfusion reactions and the rejection of transplanted organs. *B cells* produce antibodies and are particularly effective in destroying bacteria and inactivating their toxins. *NK (natural killer) cells* attack a wide variety of infectious microbes and tumorous cells. *Monocytes* (3-

8% of WBCs) have nucleus which is kidney- or horseshoe-shaped. They are rare within the circulatory system, as they soon migrate into the tissues, where they enlarge and differentiate into macrophages. Some of these cells are fixed (tissue) macrophages, like in the lungs or in the spleen, while others become wandering macrophages, which gather at sites of tissue infection or inflammation. They clean up cellular debris and microbes by phagocytosis. (Table 9.1).

Table 9.1: Significance of high and low white blood cell count.

WBC Type	*High Count May Indicate*	*Low Count May Indicate*
Neutrophils inflammation	Bacterial infection, burns, stress,	Radiation exposure, drug toxicity vitamin B12 deficiency, systemic lupus erythematosus (SLE)
Eosinophils	Allergic reactions, parasitic infections, autoimmune diseases	Drug toxicity, stress
Basophils	Allergic reactions, leukemias, cancers, hypothyroidism	Pregnancy, ovulation, stress, hyperthyroidism
Lymphocytes	Viral infections, some leukemias	Prolonged illness, immunosuppression, treatment with cortisol
Monocytes	Viral or fungal infections, tuberculosis, some leukemias, other chronic diseases	Bone marrow suppression, treatment with cortisol

Platelets are irregularly disc-shaped, 2-4 μm diameter cellular fragments of megakaryocytes. They have a short life span (4-9 days) in the circulation and then are removed by fixed macrophages in the spleen or liver. They have no nuclei but contain many vesicles which promote blood clotting upon the release of their content. Platelets additionally help stop blood loss by forming a platelet plug in the damaged vessels.

COLLECTION, SOURCES AND AMOUNT OF BLOOD SAMPLE

Since blood is confined within the cardiovascular system, the skin has to be punctured before blood can be obtained. There are two common sources of blood for routine laboratory tests: *blood from a superficial vein* by puncturing it with a needle and syringe, or *from skin capillaries* by skin-prick. Arterial blood and blood from cardiac chambers may be required for special tests (Table 9.2).

Table 9.2: Sources and Differences between Venous Blood and Capillary Blood

Venous Blood	***Capillary Blood***
1. It is obtained from a superficial vein by venepuncture	1. It is obtained from a skin puncture, usually over a finger, ear lobe/or the heal of a foot
2. A clean venepuncture provides blood without any contamination with tissue fluid	2. Blood from a skin prick comes from punctured capillaries and from smallest arterioles and venules
3. There is less risk of contamination since sterile syringe and needle are used	3. There is greater risk of contamination and transmission of disease as one may be careless about sterilization since skin prick is considered a harmless procedure
4. Cell counts, Hb, and PCV values are generally higher	4. These values are likely to be on the lower side since some tissue fluid is bound to dilute the blood even when it is free-flowing
5. Venous blood is preferable when normal blood standards are to be established, or when two samples from the same person are to be compared at different times	5. Capillary blood is not suitable for these purposes

i. ***Capillary blood***: The skin and other tissues are richly supplied with capillaries, so when a drop or a few drops of blood are required, as for estimation of Hb, cell counts, BT and CT, blood films, micro chemical tests, etc, blood from a skin puncture (skin-prick) with a lancet or needle is adequate.

ii. ***Venous blood***: When larger amounts (say, a few ml that cannot be obtained from a skin puncture) are needed as for complete hematological and biochemical investigations, venous blood is obtained with a syringe and needle by puncturing a superficial vein. In infants, venous blood may have to be taken from the femoral vein, or the frontal venous sinus.

COLLECTION OF CAPILLARY BLOOD (SKIN-PRICK METHOD)

Capillary blood is also called "peripheral blood" as it comes out of the peripheral vessels (capillaries) in contrast to venous blood.

Selection of Site for Skin Prick

In adults and older children, capillary blood is generally obtained from a skin puncture made on the tip of the middle or ring finger, or on the lobe of the ear. In infants and young children in whom the fingers are too small for a prick, the medial or lateral side of the pad of the big toe or heel is used.

The site for skin-prick should be clean and free from edema, infection, skin disease, callus, or circulatory defects.

1. ***Blood Lancet/Pricking needle*:** Disposable, sterile, one-time use, blood lancets (flat, thin metal pieces with 3–4 mm deep penetrating sharp points) are commercially available and should be preferred. Lancets with 3-sided cutting points and mounted in plastic are also suitable. However, lancets with thin and shallow points are not satisfactory. Ordinary, narrow-bore injection needles are useless since they only make shallow cuts rather than deep punctures. However, wide-bore (22 gauge) needles may be used in an emergency or if blood lancets are not available.

   A cutting needle with 3-sided cutting point (used by surgeons) can serve the purpose well.

   Pricking gun. A spring-loaded pricking gun that has a disposable, 3-sided sharp point, and a loading and releasing mechanism, is ideal because the depth of the puncture can be preselected. After pulling back the release lever, and thus "loading" the gun, it is placed on the ball of the finger and the release lever pressed. The subject does not see the sharp point and the pain is thus minimized.
2. Sterile gauze/cotton, moist with 70% alcohol/methylated spirit.
3. Glass slides, pipettes, etc. according to requirements.

PROCEDURES

All aseptic precautions must be taken. The person giving the prick should wash his/her hands with soap and water, and wear gloves if possible.

1. Clean and vigorously rub the ball of the finger with the spirit swab, followed by a final cleaning with dry gauze. (Scrubbing increases local blood flow).

   Allow the alcohol to dry by evaporation for the following reasons:

   i. Sterilization with alcohol/spirit is effective only after it has dried by evaporation.

   ii. The thin film of alcohol can cause the blood drop to spread sideways along with alcohol so that it will not form a satisfactory round drop.

   iii. The alcohol may cause hemolysis of blood.

2. Steadying the finger to be pricked in your left hand, apply a gentle pressure on the sides of the ball of the finger with your thumb and forefinger to raise a thick, broad ridge of skin. (Do not touch the pricking area).
3. Hold the lancet between the thumb and fingers of your right hand, and keeping it directed along the axis of the finger, but slightly "off" center so as to miss the tip of the phalanx (*i.e.* not too far down or too far near the top of the nail bed), prick the skin with a sharp and quick vertical stab to a depth of 3–4 mm and release the pressure. The blood should start to flow slowly, spontaneously and freely (without any squeezing)—if a good prick has been given.
4. Wipe away the first 2 drops of blood with dry, sterile gauze as it may be contaminated not only with tissue fluid, but also with epithelial and endothelial cells which will appear as artifacts in the blood film.
5. Allow a fresh drop of blood of sufficiently large size (about 3–4 mm diameter) to well up from the wound, and make a blood smear, or fill a pipette as the case may be.
6. Clean the area of the prick with a fresh swab and ask the subject to keep the swab pressed on the wound with his/her thumb till the bleeding stops, which occurs in a minute or so.

PRECAUTIONS

1. Keep the equipment for the test ready before getting/giving a finger prick

2. The selected site should be clean, free from infection, edema, or skin disease
3. The site should be vigorously cleaned and scrubbed with sterile gauze and alcohol. Scrubbing increases local blood flow
4. The lancet/needle should be sterile, and if it is to be reused, it should be passed through a flame
5. The puncture should be deep enough to give free-flowing blood but not so very deep that it takes inordinately long time for the bleeding to stop
6. Do not press or squeeze the finger to increase the blood flow from the skin-prick, though the arm or the hand may be milked towards the fingers.

Disinfect the pad of the middle finger with ethanol. Stop circulation in the middle of the finger with the thumb until the end of the middle finger has deep red colour. Press the fingerpricker on the skin of the middle finger, and press the button releasing the needle. Throw the used fingerpricker immediately into the hazardous waste! Wipe off the first drop of blood as it contains a large amount of other tissue fragments, and start drawing blood. If bleeding subsides, massage the fingers.

Experiment No. 10

Aim: Introduction to Hemocytometry

***Key words*:** Hemocytometry, Using Hemocytometer, Diluting Pipettes, Diluting Fluids, Charging the chamber, Counting pattern, Units for reporting

HEMOCYTOMETRY

Hemocytometer is the technique to count blood cells (to count WBC, RBC, and Platelets, as well as, counting cells in other body fluids, *e.g.* CSF and semen analysis) by using the hemocytometer.

Principle

Since the number of blood cells is very high, it is difficult to count them even under the microscope. This difficulty is partly overcome by diluting the blood to a known degree with suitable diluting fluids and then counting them.

The sample of blood is diluted in a special pipette and is then placed in a capillary space of known capacity (volume) between a counting chamber and a coverslip. The cells spread out in a single layer which makes their counting easy. Knowing the dilution employed, the number of cells in undiluted blood can then easily be calculated.

Hemocytometer

The hemocytometer set consists of the following:

1. ***The counting chamber*:** It is a thick glass slide, appropriately ruled with a counting grid, *i.e.* squares of varying dimensions.
2. ***The diluting pipettes*:** Two different glass capillary pipettes, each having a bulb, are provided for counting RBCs and WBCs. (These pipettes are sometimes called "cell pipettes" or blood pipettes. The third pipette that the students will be using is the hemoglobin pipette, which does not have a bulb).
3. ***Coverslips:*** Special coverslips having an optically plane and uniform surface should be preferred over ordinary coverslips.
4. *RBC and WBC* diluting fluids.

Steps in Hemocytometry

The whole process of cell counting involves the following steps:

1. Keeping all the equipment ready
2. Getting a sample of blood
3. *Pipetting and dilution, i.e.* filling the pipette with blood and diluting it
4. *Charging, i.e.* filling the counting chamber with diluted blood
5. Counting the cells and reporting the results.

The Counting Chamber

It is made of heavy glass with strict specifications, it resemble a glass slide. It is very thick and non-flexible. There are many types of hemocytometer differing from one another in rulings, but the commonest and the easiest one is the *Improved Neubauer Chamber, bright line type.*

When viewing the hemocytometer from the top (Fig.10.1a), it has 2 ruled platforms and 2 raised platforms. The ruled areas are separated by depressions on three sides. Each of these platforms has a ruled counting area marked off by precise lines etched into the glass. The raised areas and depression form "H"- letter, this "H" has two coverslip supports (raised areas) on each side which are exactly 0.1 mm higher than the ruled platforms. The coverslip

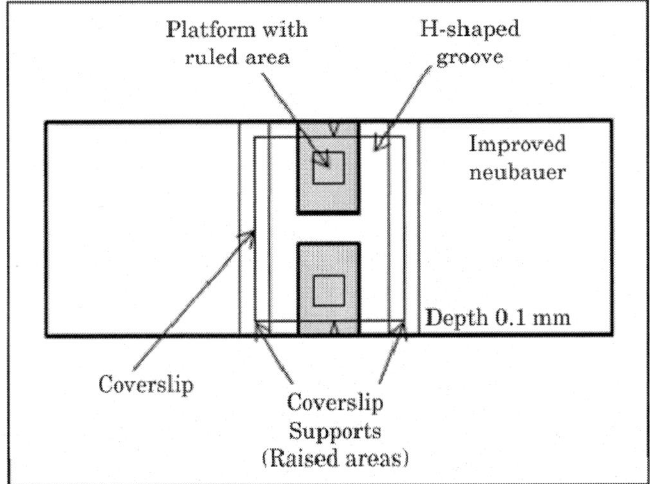

Fig. 10.1a: Top view of the Neubauer Counting Chamber

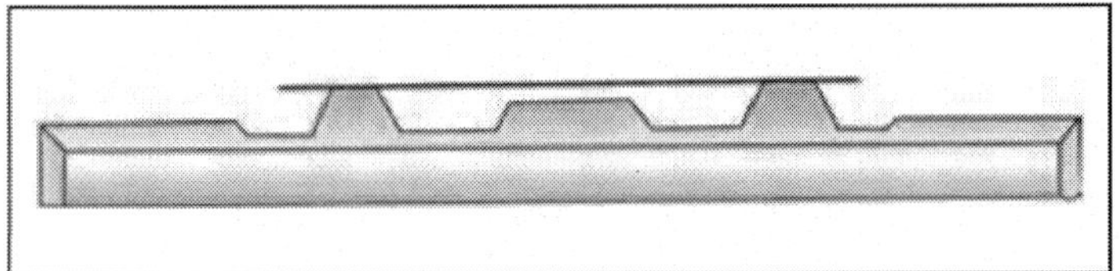

Fig. 10.1b: Coverslip position on the hemocytometer

is placed on top of the raised areas so it covers both ruled areas. The depth between the bottom of the ruled area and the coverslip is exactly 0.1 mm (Fig. 10.1b). So, coverslip function is to confine the fluid and to regulate the depth of the applied fluid.

Hemocytometer Counting Areas

Hemocytometer has 2 identical ruled counting areas, each composed of a large square, with a sides of 3 mm. This large square is subdivided to 9 small squares, each with sides of 1 mm. When cover slip is placed on raised area, each 1mm square can accommodate a volume of 1 mm x 1mm x 0.1 mm (depth) = 0.1 mm^3 (cubic millimetre). *WBC cells are counted in 4 areas of corner.*

The central square is further subdivided into 25 smaller squares each with a sides of 0.2 mm, so the volume accommodated within this square will be 0.2 mm x 0.2 mm x 0.1 mm (depth) = 0.004 mm^3 (cubic millimetre). *Red blood cells are counted in the large central square, in which only the four corner squares and the center square* (look Fig., in which "R" denotes for red blood cells).

Platelets are counted in the entire large center squares (the 25 small squares). (Fig. 10.2)

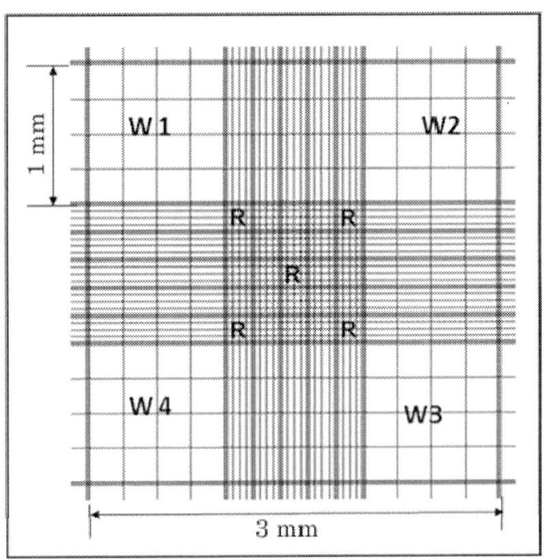

Fig. 10.2: Blood Cells Counting Area

Focusing the Counting Grid

Examine the grid on each floor piece, without the coverslip, under low and high magnifications. Move the condenser up and down, closing/adjusting the iris diaphragm at the same time. Find out the best combination of these two that shows the grid lines and squares clearly. When properly focused, the rulings (lines) appear as translucent darkish lines.

With low magnification of 100 times, one large square, 1 mm × 1 mm is visible in one field, *i.e.* a group of 16 medium squares (for WBC counting), or a groups of 25 medium squares (for RBC counting).

Examine the squares under high magnification. Compare what you see with the diagram of blood cell counting area and identify, understand, and draw the dimensions of various squares in your workbook.

Blood Cell Diluting Pipette

***Parts of a Diluting Pipette* (Table 10.1)**

***The stem*:** The long narrow stem has a capillary bore and a well-grounded conical tip. It is divided into 10 equal parts (graduations) but has only two numbers etched on it—0.5 in the middle of the stem, and 1.0 at the junction of stem and the bulb. The pipette has a glossy white surface behind the graduations to facilitate their reading. (Note that some pipettes have only two graduations—0.5 and 1.0).

Table 10.1: Difference between WBC and RBC Diluting Pipettes

Feature	*RBC Pipette*	*WBC Pipette*
1) Bead	It has a red bead	It has a white bead
2) Graduations	It has graduations up to mark 101	It has graduations up to mark 11
3) Bulb	Size of bulb is larger. The volume of the bulb is 100 times the volume contained in stem.	Size of bulb is smaller. The volume of the blub is 10 times the volume of the stem.
4) Lumen	Size of lumen is smaller. The capillary bore is narrow, thus it is a *slow-speed pipette*.	Size of lumen is larger. The capillary bore is wider; hence it is a *fast-speed pipette.*
5) Mouth Piece	Red	White
6) Dilution	The dilution can be 1 in 200.	The dilution can be 1 in 20.

***The bulb*:** The stem widens into a bulb which contains a free-rolling bead—red in the RBC pipette, Fig. 10.4 and white in the WBC pipette Fig. 10.3. The bead helps in mixing the blood and the diluent and also helps in quick identification at a glance.

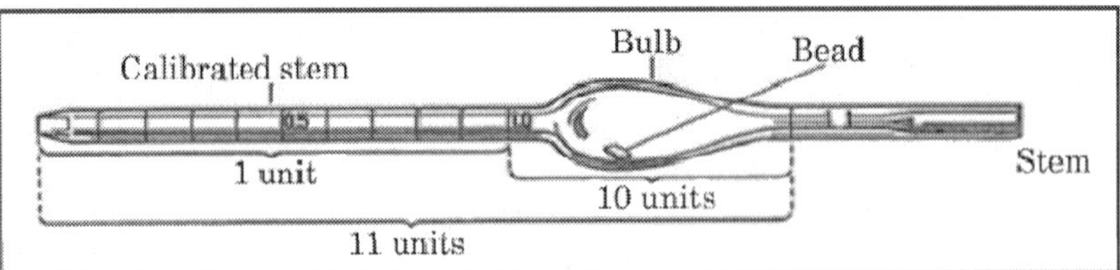

Fig. 10.3: White blood cell diluting pipette

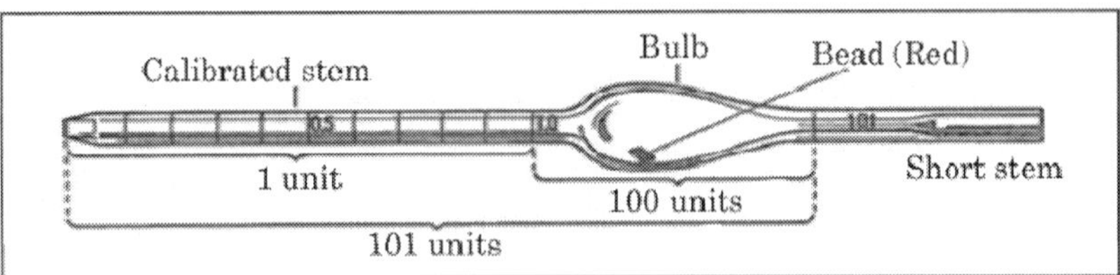

Fig. 10.4: Red blood cell diluting pipette

Rubber Tube and Mouthpiece

The bulb narrows again into a short stem to which a long, narrow, soft-rubber tube bearing a mouthpiece (often white in WBC pipette Fig. 10.3 and red in RBC pipette Fig. 10.4) is attached. The rubber tube should be at least 25–30 cm long to facilitate filling of the pipette by gentle suction. It also allows the pipette to be held horizontally so that one can comfortably watch the blood or diluting fluid entering the pipette.

Just beyond the bulb, the number 101 is etched on the RBC, and 11 on the WBC pipettes.

Calculation of Dilution Obtained (Dilution Factor)

When blood is sucked up to the mark 0.5 (half part or volume) and is followed by the diluting fluid, the blood enters the bulb first and is followed by the diluent to the mark 101 (RBC pipette), or mark 11 (WBC pipette). The stem in both pipettes contains only the diluent. Thus, *the dilution of the blood occurs in the bulb only.*

RBC pipette: Since the volume of the bulb is 100 (101 – 1.0 = 100), it means that 100 volumes (or parts) of diluted blood contain 0.5 (half) part of blood and 99.5 (100 – 0.5 = 99.5) parts or volumes of diluent. This gives a dilution of 0.5 in 100 (half in hundred), or 1 in 200 (one in two hundred); *i.e.* 1 part blood, and 199 parts of diluent, or 200 times. This figure of 200 is called *the dilution factor.*

***WBC pipette*:** In this case the volume of the bulb is 10 (11 – 1 = 10). When blood is taken to the mark 0.5 (half part or volume) followed by diluent to the mark 11, the volume of the diluted blood is now 10, which contains 0.5 part blood and 9.5 parts or volumes of the diluting fluid. This gives a dilution of 0.5 in 10 (half in ten), or 1 in 20 (one in twenty), the dilution factor being 20 (the blood will be diluted 20 times).

Precautions for Using Diluting Pipette

1. The pipette should be clean and dry and the bead should roll freely.
2. While filling the pipette with blood, it should not be lifted out of the blood drop, otherwise air will enter it.
3. Once the blood has been taken in the stem, drawing up of diluents should not be delayed, otherwise it will clot in it.
4. The pipette should be cleaned soon after the experiment is over.

Using the Hemocytometer

Position a clean, dust free, coverslip so it covers the ruled counting areas of a clean hemocytometer. Place the hemocytometer on the microscope stage, so one of the ruled counting areas is aligned directly above the light source (condenser); rotate the low power objective (x10) into place; using the coarse focus knob, move the low power objective very near the coverslip; rotate coarse focus knob to increase the distance between the low power objective (X10) and the hemocytometer until ruled lines come into focus; all nine large squares must be viewable; very carefully, rotate the high power objective (X45) into place, with the aid of fine focus knob, adjust the focus until the etched lines come into focus, you can now carefully move the hemocytometer by using the mechanical stage, so that the ruled area on the other side can be viewed.

Fill the hemacytometer with the fluid containing cells to be counted, by touching the micropipette tip to the point where the coverslip and raised platform meet on one side, the fluid will drawn under the coverslip and over the counting area by capillary action. The chamber must not be overfilled or underfilled, if accurate results are needed.

Charging the Counting Chamber

Charging the chamber requires patience, practice, and understanding of how to correctly judge the size of the drop, the angle at which the pipette should be held and the time needed for filling (charging) the chamber. This is called the "speed of the pipette". Obviously, it varies with the size of the capillary bore in the stem of the pipette.

High-speed pipette

Since the bore of the WBC pipette is wider, a drop will form more quickly at its tip, and it will be larger, as compared to the RBC pipette. This requires that the WBC pipette should be held more horizontally at an angle of 20–30° and for a shorter time.

Slow-speed pipette

The bore of the RBC pipette being narrow, it will take a longer time for a suit-able drop to form. It should, therefore, be held at a steeper angle say, 40–60°.

It is for this reason that the students should first practice charging a chamber with the RBC pipette and then with the WBC pipette.

Ideally-charged chamber

An ideally-charged chamber is completely filled with diluted blood. If any blood flows into the grooves, it is called "*overcharging*". If the fluid is insufficient to cover the floor piece, or if there are air bubbles, it is called "*undercharging*", (air bubbles are formed if the coverslip or the floor piece is dirty with grease or is moist).

Precautions

1. Ensure that the counting chamber and the coverslip are absolutely clean, grease-free, and dry.
2. While charging the chamber ensure that it is neither under nor over-charged.
3. Never bring the objective lens down while looking into the microscope as the chamber is likely to be scratched or broken.

If there is over or under-charging, wash the chamber and coverslip in soap and water, dry them and recharge the chamber.

Once the chamber has been properly charged, wait for 2–3 minutes so that the cells settle down. Counting cannot be started when the cells are moving and changing places due to currents in the fluid.

The Counting Pattern

Either left to right or right to left counting pattern can be used (Fig. 10.5 and Fig. 10.6); but with the insurance that each cell is counted only once, to accomplish this, cells that touch the right boundary lines or the bottom boundary lines are not counted, because they will be counted with the other squares (look figure). After cells are counted on one side, the hemocytometer is moved and the cells are counted on the other side. Results for each side are recorded, then are totaled and calculated.

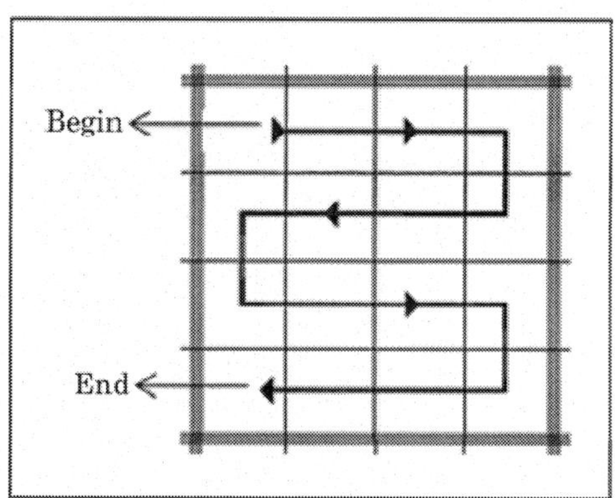

Fig. 10.5 Counting Pattern

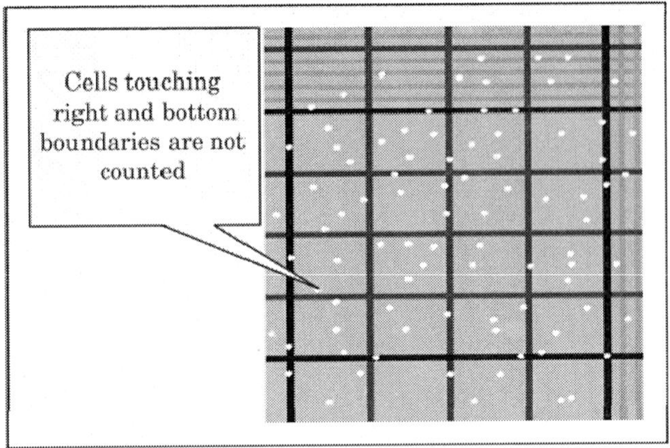

Fig. 10.6: Cells touching the right and bottom boundaries are not counted

Rules for Counting

i. Cells lying within a square are to be counted with that square.
ii. Cells lying on or touching its upper horizontal and left vertical lines are to be counted with that particular square.

Units for Reporting

The result of cell counting is usually expressed as "................ cells per cubic millimetre (cumm; mm^3; µl) of blood". For example, RBC count = 5.0 million RBCs/cumm.

The SI unit, however, is ....cells per litre of blood. 1 mm^3 = 1 µl = 10^{-6} litre, 1 µl × 10^6 = 1 litre

QUESTIONS

Q. What is the principle underlying the use of a counting chamber?

Q. What are the dimensions of WBC and RBC squares?

Q. What are the features of an ideally-charged chamber?

Q. How will you identify a red cell pipette and *a white cell pipette?*

Q. What is the function of the bead in the bulb?
The bead helps to mix the blood with its diluent. It tells whether the pipette is dry or not. (It rolls freely if it is dry.) It also helps to identify the pipette by just glancing at it.

Q. What are the units of markings on the pipettes?
There are no absolute units of volume marked on the pipette. They only denote relative volumes or parts in relation to each other.

Q. What is the function of the bulb in a diluting pipette?
The dilution of the blood occurs in the bulb only, and since the volume of the bulb is known, it is possible to dilute the blood with a diluent in accurately known proportions.

Q. Why is it important to discard the first two-three drops of diluted blood from the pipette before charging the counting chamber?
After the blood has been diluted in the pipette, the stem contains only the cell-free diluent. This fluid has, therefore, to be discarded before the chamber can be filled.

Q. How will you clean a pipette when blood has clotted in the stem?
The pipette is kept in strong nitric acid for 24 hours. A flexible suitably thick metal wire is used to clean the capillary bore after washing the pipette in running water. The process may have to be repeated.

Q. Can a pipette be used for any other purpose than cell counting?
The RBC pipette can be used for counting platelets, WBCs (when their number is very high, as in some leukemias) or spermatozoa in the semen.

Q. What is the principle underlying the use of a counting chamber?

Q. What are the dimensions of WBC and RBC squares?

Q. What are the features of an ideally-charged chamber?

Q. How does the improved Neubauer chamber differ from the older variety of Neubauer chamber?

Experiment No. 11

Aim: To Determine Total Leukocyte Count (TLC)

***Key words*:** WBC, Types, Formation, Turk's fluid, Disorders

WHITE CELL COUNT (WCC)

The white blood cells (WBCs; leukocytes) are the *mobile units* constitute the major defense system of the body against invasion by bacteria, viruses, fungi, toxins and other foreign invaders. Their number is kept remarkably constant in health, but it increases or decreases in many diseases, particularly acute and chronic infections.

They are formed partially in the bone marrow Fig. 11.1 (*granulocytes* and *monocytes* and a few *lymphocytes*) and partially in the lymph tissue (*lymphocytes* and *plasma cells*). After formation, they are transported in the blood to different parts of the body where they are needed. The real value of the white blood cells is that most of them are specifically transported to areas of serious infection and inflammation, thereby providing a rapid and potent defense against infectious agents. As we see later, the granulocytes and monocytes have a special ability to "seek out and destroy" a foreign invader.

General Characteristics of Leukocytes

Types of White Blood Cells Six types of white blood cells are normally present in the blood. They are *polymorphonuclear neutrophils, polymorphonuclear eosinophils, polymorphonuclear basophils, monocytes, lymphocytes,* and, occasionally, *plasma cells*. In addition,

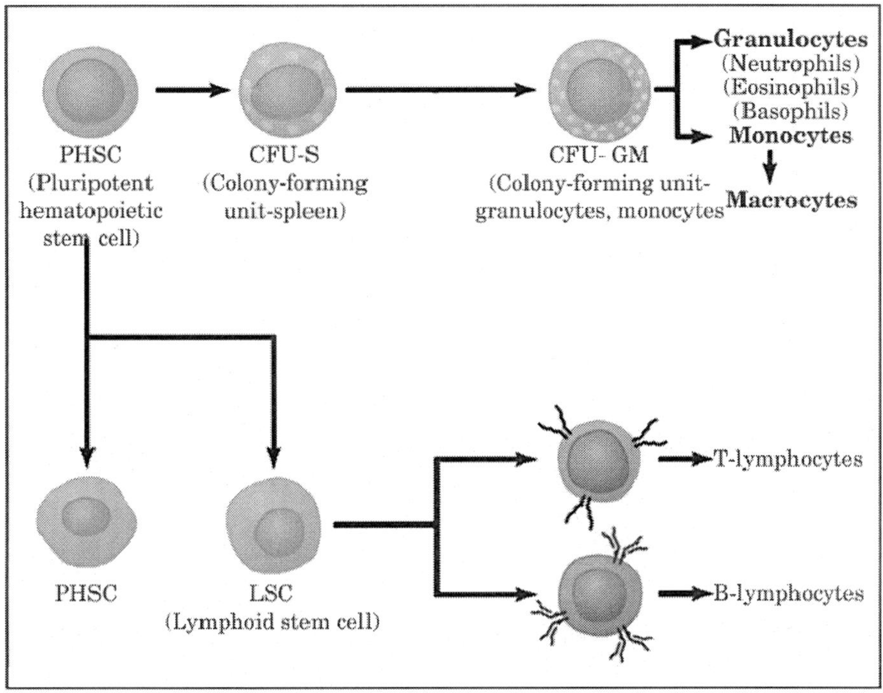

Fig. 11.1: Formation of Leukocytes

there are large numbers of *platelets,* which are fragments of another type of cell similar to the white blood cells found in the bone marrow, the *megakaryocyte*. The first three types of cells, the polymorphonuclear cells, all have a granular appearance.

Normal Values

White blood cell count:

$4000 - 11000$ cells/ mm^3 or

$4.0 - 11.0 \times 10^3$ cells/ μL

Note:

$1\mu L = 1\ mm^3 = 10^{-6}$ litre.

Principle

WBC count or TLC is defined as the total numbers of WBCs per unit volume (mm^3 or μL) of undiluted blood. As the numbers of leukocytes are high and their size is small, it is difficult to count the cells even under high power objective. To overcome this difficulty, whole blood is diluted with appropriate diluting fluid to a known degree (1:20). Dilution of blood sample destroys the red cells and stains the nuclei of the leukocytes. This diluted sample is then placed inside the capillary space made by the counting chamber and cover glass allowing the cells to be spread in single layer on counting grid. Cells are counted in four corner areas of counting chamber using low power objective (10X) and their number in undiluted blood reported as leukocytes/mm^3.

APPARATUS AND MATERIALS

1. ***Microscope*:** Counting chamber (Preferably, Improved Neubauer Chamber) with a coverslip. Blood lancet/pricking needle. •Sterile cotton/gauze swabs. •70% alcohol.
2. ***WBC pipette*:** White bead in bulb, and markings 0.5, 1.0, and 11.
3. ***White cell diluting fluid or Turk's fluid*:** This fluid is used for diluting the blood specimen for WBC count. Turk's fluid hemolyses RBCs due to acidity and stains the nuclei of WBCs as it contains the dye, so that counting of leukocytes can be done with ease. (Table 11.1).

Table 11.1: Composition of Turk's solution

Ingredients	*Quantity*	*Purpose*
Glacial acetic acid	2.0 mL	Hemolyzes RBCs without affecting WBCs
Gentian violet (1% Aqueous Solution)	1.0 mL	Stains the nuclei of WBCs
Distilled water (q.s.)	100 mL	As diluent

Note: Methylene blue (1 mL of 0.3% solution in water, w/v) can be used in place of Gentian violet. Small quantity of thymol may be added to the dilution fluid to prevent growth of moulds.

Procedures

1. Collect all the requirements. Clean and dry them carefully.
2. Place the counting chamber on the microscope stage with coverslip. Adjust the illumination, and focus the WBC

Counting area. There are 4 corner squares each of 1 mm^2 area. Each corner square is further divided into 16 smaller squares. You will see all the squares in one field.

3. Observing all the aseptic precautions, get a finger-prick, discard the first drop of blood, and allow the next good-sized drop to form.
4. ***Filling the pipette*:** Dip the tip of the pipette in the edge of the drop, draw blood to the 0.5 mark. Wipe off the excess blood from tip and sides of the pipette and suck Turk's fluid to the mark 11. Mix the contents of the bulb thoroughly for 3–4 minutes (Fig. 11.2).
5. ***Charging the chamber*:** Discard the first 2–3 drops of fluid from the pipette and charge the chamber. The chamber should neither be over-charged nor under-charged.
6. Allow the cells to settle for 3–4 minutes. Use the fine adjustment again and try to identify the WBCs under low magnification. The leukocytes appear as round, shiny (refractile), darkish dots, with a halo around them. These 'dots' represent the nuclei, which have been stained by gentian violet. The cytoplasm is not stained. Do not confuse with dust particles which have varying sizes and shapes, often angular. They are usually opaque, with no 'halo' around them. They may be brown, black or yellow in color.

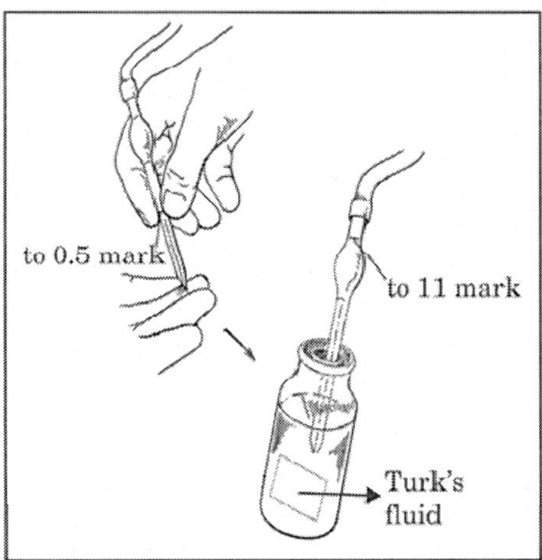

Fig. 11.2: Filling the pipette and diluting the blood sample

7. ***Counting the cells:*** Count the cells under low power lens.

   Count the WBCs in 16 squares under low power. Count the cells in the 4 groups of 16 squares Each, *i.e.,* in a total of 64 squares. Draw appropriate squares in your work-book for entering the counts. As follows:

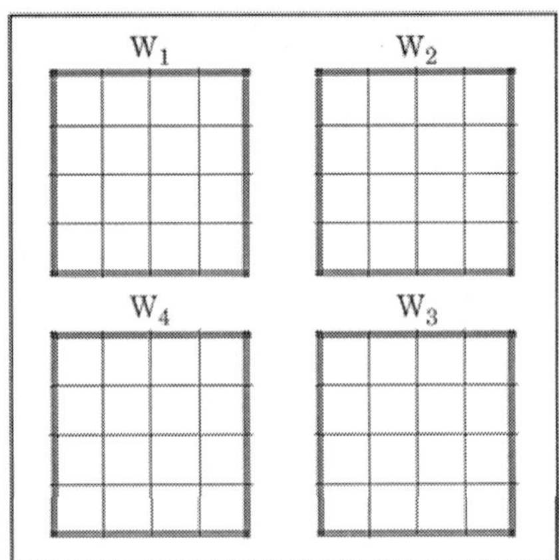

Calculations

1. *Total cells counted in 4 W sections* = $W_1 + W_2 + W_3 + W_4$
2. *Dilution correction factor*

   We have diluted 0.5 part of blood by 10 parts of dilution fluid i.e.

   $$0.5 \rightarrow 10$$
   $$\therefore 1.0 \rightarrow 20$$

   Hence, Dilution correction factor is 20
3. *Volume correction factor*

   a) Area of 1 W section is = 1 mm^2.

   But, we have used 4 W sections for counting WBCs,

   $$\therefore \text{Total area of 4 W sections} = 1 mm^2 \times 4 = 4 mm^2$$

   b) Total volume of 4 W sections = Total area of 4 W sections × Depth = 4 mm^2 × 0.1 mm = 0.4 mm^3

This means, we have counted cells in 0.4 mm^3 volume. But Total Leukocyte Count (TLC) is defined as the total numbers of leukocytes per cumm (mm^3) or per microlitre (µL) of undiluted blood.

Hence, Volume correction is required.

$$\therefore \text{Volume Correction factor} = \frac{\text{Volume desired}}{\text{Volume used}} = \frac{1}{0.4}$$

Therefore, volume correction factor is 2.5

4. *Total leukocyte count* = Total cells counted in 4 W sections × Dilution Correction Factor × Volume Correction Factor

$$= \chi \times 20 \times 2.5$$
$$= \chi \times 50$$

Therefore, TLC = ______________WBCs/ mm^3 of blood

Precautions

1. Keep all equipment ready before getting a prick.
2. WBC Pipette and Neubauer chamber should be dry thoroughly.
3. Wipe off first drop of blood as it contains tissue fluid.
4. Pipette is filled by blood exactly upto 0.5 mark. If it is taken beyond this mark, tap the pipette against the palm gently.
5. Wipe off the tip of pipette before sucking diluting fluid.
6. Blood in the pipette must be diluted quickly to avoid clotting of blood and clogging of pipette. Suck the dilution fluid upto 11 mark exactly. If it exceeds the mark, repeat the procedure.
7. When mixing the blood with the Turk's fluid, give sufficient time for complete hemolysis of red cells. However, ensure that the leukocytes are not centrifuged towards the ends of the pipette which can be avoided by keeping the pipette horizontal while mixing the contents of the bulb.
8. Overcharging and undercharging of the chamber must be avoided. Though the condition of a charged chamber may

remain stable for 80–90 minutes, the count is usually stable for 30–40 minutes. After that, the diluted blood starts receding due to drying and the count decreases. The counting of the cells should, therefore, not be delayed.

9. To avoid counting of the same cells twice, counting rules and counting pattern must be followed

Results and Conclusion

Total leukocyte count (TLC) of own blood is ____________ *cells / mm^3 or* _____ *×10^3 cells / μL.*

Normal count: 4000 - 11000 cells/mm^3 or 4.0 - 11.0 ×10^3 cells/μL

Therefore the count is *Increased / Decreased* indicating *Leukocytosis / Leukopenia*.

DISCUSSION

Leukocytosis

The term refers to an increase in the number of WBCs beyond 11000/mm^3 irrespective of the type of cells (granulocytes, monocytes, lymphocytes, etc.) that are involved in raising TLC. Thus, unless mentioned otherwise (*e.g.*, lymphocytosis, eosinophilia, etc.), the term refers to an increase in the number of neutrophils, the commonest cause of a raised TLC. The terms leukocytosis, granulocytosis, and neutrophilia, are more or less synonymous.

Leukocytosis is a normal, protective response of the body to various types of stresses, such as infections, severe exercise, surgery, tissue injury, etc.

Physiological Leukocytosis

About 95% of the people have a TLC within the normal range. Physiological leukocytosis (*i.e.*, in the absence of infection or tissue injury) has no clinical significance. There is no decrease or absence of eosinophils (eosinopenia), which is a feature of leukocytosis due to infection. Physiological leukocytosis is due to mobilization of WBCs from the marginal pool or bone marrow reserve ("Shift" leukocytosis). It is seen in the following conditions:

1. *Normal infants*: The count may be as high as 18–20,000/mm^3 but it returns to normal level within 1–2 years.
2. *Food intake and digestion ("digestive leukocytosis")*: There is a mild increase which returns to normal within an hour or so.
3. *Physical exercise.*
4. *Mental stress.*
5. *Pregnancy:* The count may be quite high, especially during the first pregnancy.
6. *Parturition*: The high TLC is possibly due to tissue injury, pain, physical stress, and hemorrhage.
7. *Extremes of temperatures*: Exposure to sun or to very low temperature can increase the WBC count.

Pathological Leukocytosis

A rise in TLC in disease is seen in:

1. *Acute infection with pyogenic (pus forming) bacteria:* The infection (due to cocci bacteria streptococcus, staphylococcus) may be:
   a. Localized, such as boils, abscess, tonsillitis, appendicitis, etc.
   b. Generalized, such as in septicemia and pyemia, bronchitis, pneumonia, peritonitis, meningitis, etc.
2. *Myocardial infarction*: The rise in TLC due to tissue injury is not seen immediately after a heart attack but only after 4–5 days.
3. *Acute hemorrhage:* Maximum response occurs in 8–10 hours, the count returning to normal in 5–6 days.
4. *Burns*: Maximum response occurs in 5–15 hours, the count returning to normal in 2–3 days.
5. Amoebic hepatitis.

6. *Malignancies*: High counts are seen in half the cases; secondary infection enhances the count.
7. *Surgical operations*: A postoperative rise is seen in all cases.

Leukopenia

The term refers to a decrease in the number of white cells (usually granulocytes; granulocytopenia) below the normal lower limit of $4000/mm^3$.

Physiological Leukopenia

A decrease in TLC under normal physiological conditions is unusual and rare. Exposure to extreme cold, even under arctic conditions and in spite of acclimatization, may reduce the count to only slightly below the $4000/mm^3$ level.

Pathological Leukopenia

Leukopenia due to disease, where TLC is abnormally low, is never beneficial to the body. In fact, it may endanger the life of the patient. The condition is almost always due to a decrease in neutrophils (neutropenia) and may be caused by various drugs used in treatment, radiation, or certain infections as described below.

1. *Infection with non-pyogenic organisms:* Typhoid and paratyphoid fevers, and sometimes in protozoal infection like malaria.
2. *Viral infections:* Influenza, mumps, smallpox, AIDS (Acquired immunodeficiency syndrome).
3. *Drugs:* Chloramphenicol, sulphonamides, aspirin, penicillins, cyclosporins, phenytoin, etc. Cytotoxic drugs used in treating malignancies may also cause leukopenis by depressing the bone marrow (other blood cells may also decrease).
4. *Repeated exposures to X-rays and radium:* These are used as radiotherapy in cancers, and cause bone marrow depression.
5. *Chemical poisons that depress bone marrow:* Arsenic, dinitrophenol, antimony and others.

6. *Malnutrition:* Deficiency of vitamin B_{12} and folate, general malnutrition, starvation, extreme weakness and debility.
7. *Hypoplasia and aplasia:* Partial or complete depression of bone marrow, *i.e.,* failure of stem cells, may occur as a result of autoimmunity, and other factors.

Leukemias

It is a group of malignant neoplasms (new growths) of WBC forming organs bone marrow and lymphoid tissue. There is an uncontrolled production and release of mature and immature WBCs into the circulation. The leukemias (commonly called blood cancers) may be myeloid (usually involving neutrophils) or lymphatic (involving lymphocytes), and acute or chronic.

Table11.2: Terminology used for abnormalities of Leukocytes

Term	*Meaning*
Leucocytosis	Increased white cell count
Neutrophilia (or neutrophil leucocytosis)	Increased neutrophil count
Lymphocytosis	Increased lymphocyte count
Monocytosis	Increased monocyte count
Eosinophilia	Increased eosinophil count
Basophilia	Increased basophil count
Thrombocytosis	Increased platelet count
Leucopenia	Decreased white cell count
Neutropenia	Decreased neutrophil count
Lymphopenia (or lymphocytopenia)	Decreased lymphocyte count
Monocytopenia	Decreased monocyte count
Eosinopenia	Decreased eosinophil count
Basopenia	Decreased basophil count

QUESTIONS

Q. What is the composition of Turk's fluid? What is the function of each constituent?

The diluting fluid for TLC contains glacial acetic acid, gentian violet and distilled water. The acid hemolyzes the red cells, without affecting the WBCs at this concentration. The dye stains the nuclei of leukocytes.

Q. What is meant by the term 'glacial'? Why should the acid in the 'Turk's fluid be glacial?

The term glacial means pure acetic acid. Only the glacial acid can give the typical 'shine' (halo) or clear refractility around the WBCs due to swelling of nuclei. This differentiates them from dust particles which are opaque and of different shapes. (It is called glacial because during its manufacture, it gives the appearance of a glacier at one stage).

Q. Why are the red cells not seen when counting the leukocytes?

The red cells are not seen because they are hemolyzed by the acid.

Q. What is the normal total leukocyte count?

The normal count in adults ranges between 4000/mm^3 and 11,000/mm^3, with an average of 7000/mm^3. The count after birth may be as high as 18,000 to 20,000/mm^3, the normal levels being reached in a few years. In the adults, about 55 to 75% of the WBCs are granulocytes, while in young children, lymphocytes dominate.

Experiment No. 12

Aim: To Study Total Erythrocyte Count

***Key words*:** RBC, Erythropoiesis, Hayem's fluid, Gower's solution,

ERYTHROCYTES

The red blood cells (RBCs) are also known as the *erythrocytes*. The major function of *erythrocytes* is to transport *hemoglobin,* which in turn carries oxygen from the lungs to the tissues. Their number is kept remarkably constant in health, but it increases or decreases in many diseases, particularly acute and chronic infections. The red blood cells have other functions besides transport of hemoglobin. For instance, they contain a large quantity of *carbonic anhydrase,* an enzyme that catalyzes the reversible reaction between carbon dioxide (CO_2) and water to form carbonic acid (H_2CO_3), increasing the rate of this reaction several thousand fold. The rapidity of this reaction makes it possible for the water of the blood to transport enormous quantities of CO_2 in the form of bicarbonate ion (HCO_3^-) from the tissues to the lungs, where it is reconverted to CO_2 and expelled into the atmosphere as a body waste product. The hemoglobin in the cells is an excellent *acid-base buffer* so that the red blood cells are responsible for most of the acid-base buffering power of whole blood.

Normal RBCs, as shown in Fig. 12.1 are biconcave discs having a mean diameter of about 7.8 μM and a thickness of 2.5 μM at the thickest point and 1.0 μM or less in the center. The average volume of the red blood cell is 90 to 95 μM^3. Erythrocytes can change shapes remarkably by virtue of strong and flexible plasma membrane,

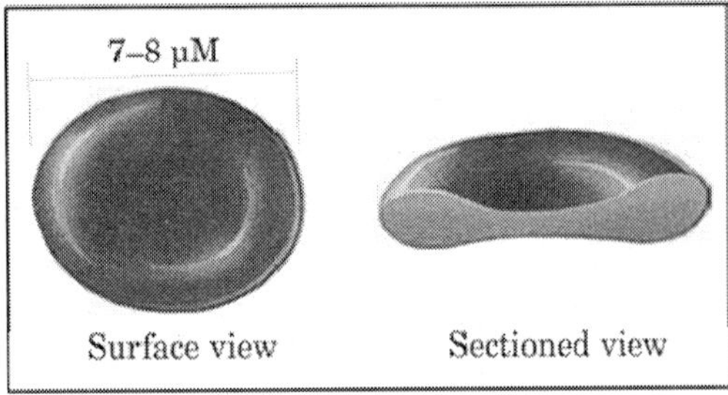

Fig. 12.1: RBC Shape

which allows them to deform without rupturing as they squeeze through narrow capillaries.

Certain glycolipids in the plasma membrane of RBCs are antigens that account for the various blood groups such as the ABO and Rh groups. RBCs lack a nucleus and other organelles and can neither reproduce nor carry on extensive metabolic activities. The cytosol of RBCs contains hemoglobin molecules; these important molecules are synthesized before loss of the nucleus during RBC production and constitute about 33% of the cell's weight (Fig. 12.2).

Normal Values

Red blood cell count: Female: 4.2 –5.4 million cells/mm^3 or 4.2 –5.4 × 10^{-6} cells/ μL

Male: 4.7 –6.1 million cells/mm^3 or 4.7 – 6.1 × 10^{-6} cells/ μL

Note: 1 μL = 1 mm^3 = 10^{-6} liter.

Principle

Erythrocyte count is defined as the total numbers of RBCs per unit volume (mm^3 or μL) of undiluted blood. The blood is diluted 200 times in a red cell pipette and the cells are counted in the counting chamber. As the numbers of erythrocytes are high and their size is small, it is difficult to count the cells even under high power objective. To overcome this difficulty, whole blood is diluted with appropriate diluting fluid to a known degree (1:200). This diluted sample is then placed inside the capillary space made by

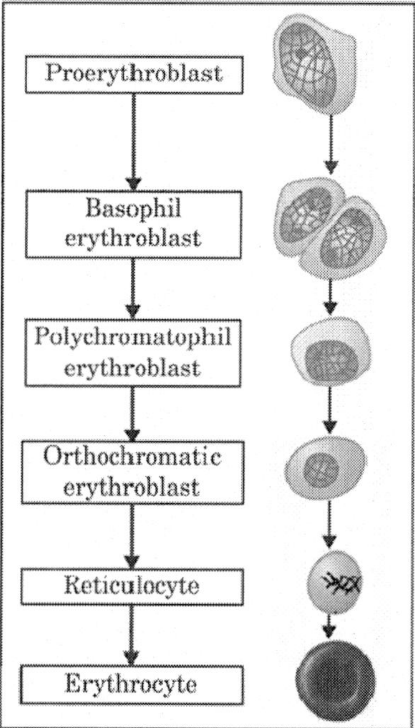

Fig. 12.2: Formation of Erythrocytes

the counting chamber and cover glass allowing the cells to be spread in single layer on counting grid. Cells are counted in four corner areas and one center area (5 R) of the central square of counting chamber by using high power objective (45X) and their number in undiluted blood reported as erythrocytes/mm^3.

APPARATUS AND MATERIALS

1. ***Microscope***: Counting chamber (Preferably, Improved Neubauer Chamber) with a coverslip. •Blood lancet/pricking needle. •Sterile cotton/gauze swabs. •70% alcohol.
2. ***RBC pipette***: Red bead in bulb, and markings 0.5, 1.0, and 101.
3. ***Red cell diluting fluid***: The ideal fluid for diluting the blood should be isotonic and neither cause hemolysis nor crenation of red cells. It should have a fixative to preserve the shape of RBCs and also prevent their autolysis so that they could be

counted even several hours after diluting the blood if necessary. It should prevent agglutination and not get spoiled on keeping. Red cell diluting fluid must be anticoagulant, antihemolytic, antiaggregation, anti-Rouleaux and preserve RBC shape. All these properties are found in Hayem's fluid (Table 12.1).

Table 12.1: Composition of Red cell diluting fluids

	Hayem's Fluid	
Ingredients	***Quantity***	***Purpose***
Sodium chloride (NaCl)	0.50 g	Sodium chloride and sodium sulfate provide isotonicity so that the red cells remain suspended in diluted blood without changing their shape and Size.
Sodium sulphate (Na_2SO_4)	2.50 g	Sodium sulphate also acts as an an anticoagulant, and as a fixative to preserve their shape and to prevent rouleaux formation (piling together of red cells)
Mercuric chloride ($HgCl_2$)	0.25 g	Mercuric chloride acts as an antifungal and anti-microbial agent and prevents contamination and growth of microorganisms.
Distilled water	100 ml	Diluent
	Gower's solution	
Sodium Sulphate	12.5 g.	Anticoagulant, and as a fixative to preserve their shape and to prevent rouleaux formation
Glacial acetic acid	33.3 ml	
Distilled water	100 ml	Diluent

Composition of Red Cell Diluting Fluids

The red blood cell diluting fluids can be used in Table 12.1

Procedures

1. Collect all the requirements. Clean and dry them carefully.
2. Place the counting chamber on the microscope stage with coverslip. Adjust the illumination, and focus the RBC Counting area, first at low power objective (10X) to observe

central counting grid. Switch the high power objective (45X) without moving the coarse adjustment knob and clear the image by fine adjustment. There are 25 squares (each with 0.04 mm^2 area) in Central Square (1 mm^2). Each of these squares is further divided into 16 smaller squares. Out of these 25 squares, four corner and one centre squares are used for RBC count.

3. Observing all the aseptic precautions, get a finger-prick, discard the first drop of blood, and allow the next good-sized drop to form.

1. ***Filling the pipette*:** Dip the tip of the pipette in the edge of the drop, draw blood to the 0.5 mark. Wipe off the excess blood from tip and sides of the pipette and suck dilution fluid up to the mark 101. Mix the contents of the bulb thoroughly for 3–4 minutes (Fig. 12.3).

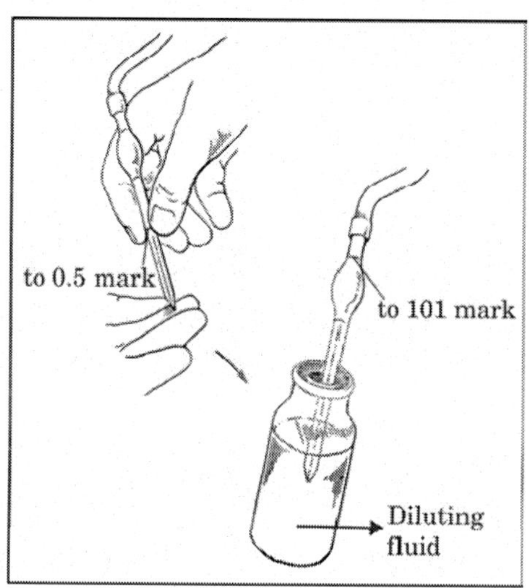

Fig. 12.3: Filling the pipette and diluting blood sample

2. ***Charging the chamber*:** Discard the first 2-3 drops of fluid from the pipette and charge the chamber. The chamber should neither be over-charged nor under-charged. Since the RBC pipette is a slow-speed pipette, it needs to be kept at an angle of 70–80° while charging the chamber.

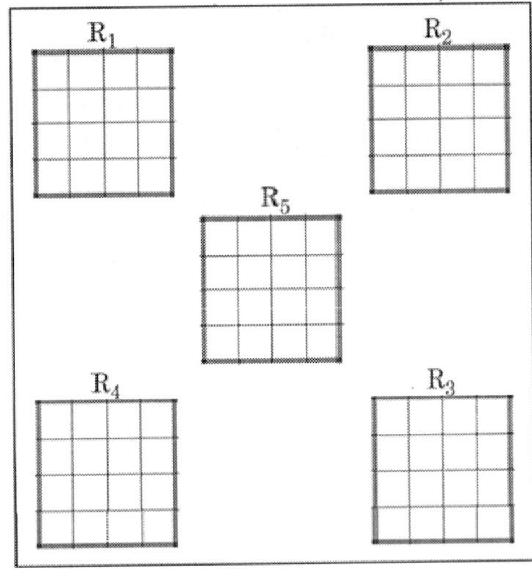

3. Allow the cells to settle for 3–4 minutes. Move the chamber carefully and bring the left upper corner block of 16 smallest squares in the field of view. (There are no smallest squares above and to its left). Use the fine adjustment again to observe the RBCs under high magnification (45×).
4. ***Counting the cells:*** Count the cells under high power lens. Count the RBCs in 16 squares under high power lens. Count the cells in the 5 groups of 16 squares each, *i.e.*, in a total of 80 squares. Draw appropriate squares in your work-book for entering the counts. As follows:

Calculations

1. ***Total cells counted in 5 R sections*** = $R_1 + R_2 + R_3 + R_4 + R_5$
2. ***Dilution Correction Factor:***

   We have diluted 0.5 part of blood by 100 parts of dilution fluid *i.e.*

   1. $0.5 \rightarrow 100$

   $\therefore 1.0 \rightarrow 200$

   Hence, Dilution correction factor is 200
3. ***Volume correction factor:***

a) Area of 1 R section is = 1/25 mm^2

= 0.04 mm^2

But, we have used 5 R sections for counting RBCs,

$\therefore$ Total area of 5 R sections = 0.04 $mm^2 \times 5$

= 0.2 mm^2

b) Total Volume of 4 W sections = Total area of 5 R sections × Depth

$$= 0.2\ mm^2 \times 0.1 mm$$
$$= 0.02\ mm^3$$

This means, we have counted cells in 0.02 mm^3 volume. But Total Erythrocyte Count is defined as the total numbers of erythrocytes per cumm (mm^3) or per microlitre (µL) of undiluted blood.

Hence, Volume correction is required.

$$\text{Volume Correction factor} = \frac{\text{Volume desired}}{\text{Volume used}}$$
$$= \frac{1}{0.02}$$
$$= 50$$

Therefore, volume correction factor is 50

4. ***Total Erythrocyte Count*** = Total cells counted in 5 R sections × Dilution Correction Factor

× Volume correction factor

$$= \chi \times 200 \times 50$$
$$= \chi \times 10000$$

Therefore, Total Erythrocyte Count = ______________RBCs/ mm^3 of blood

Precautions

1. Keep all equipment ready before getting a prick.
2. RBC Pipette and Neubauer chamber should be dry thoroughly.

3. Wipe off first drop of blood as it contains tissue fluid.
4. Pipette is filled by blood exactly upto 0.5 mark. If it is taken beyond this mark, tap the pipette against the palm gently.
5. Wipe off the tip of pipette before sucking diluting fluid.
6. Blood in the pipette must be diluted quickly to avoid clotting of blood and clogging of pipette. Suck the dilution fluid upto 101 mark exactly. If it exceeds the mark, repeat the procedure.
7. When mixing the blood with the dilution fluid, keep the pipette horizontal while mixing the contents of the bulb.
8. Overcharging and undercharging of the chamber must be avoided. Though the condition of a charged chamber may remain stable for 80–90 minutes, the count is usually stable for 30–40 minutes. After that, the diluted blood starts receding due to drying and the count decreases. The counting of the cells should, therefore, not be delayed.
9. To avoid counting of the same cells twice, counting rules and counting pattern must be followed

RESULTS AND CONCLUSION

Total Erythrocyte Count of own blood is ______________cells/mm^3 or______ million cells/ µL.

***Normal count*:** Female: 4.2 –5.4 million cells/mm^3 or 4.2 –5.4 $\times 10^{-6}$ cells/ µL

Male: 4.7 –6.1 million cells/mm^3 or 4.7 – 6.1 $\times 10^{-6}$ cells/ µL

QUESTIONS

Q.1 When blood is taken to the mark 0.5 and the diluent to mark 101, why is the dilution 1 in 200 and not 1 in 202?

Long stem of RBC diluting pipette is having 1.0 mark. When diluting fluid is sucked into the pipette the blood sample comes to the bulb where actual dilution of the blood occurs. At this moment the long arm only consists of dilution fluid and not the blood. Therefore 101 (Volume of bulb) – 1.0 (long stem) = 100. Hence, half volume in hundred gives a dilution of 1 in 200.

Q.2 Why is blood diluted 200 times for red cell count?

As the number of RBCs is very high, a high degree of dilution is required.

Q.3 What is the function of the bead in the bulb?

The bead (red in this case) helps in mixing the contents of the bulb thoroughly. It helps in identifying the pipette at a distance. And, thirdly, it tells whether the bulb is dry or not (If it is not, the bead will not roll freely).

Q.4 Which are the other dilution fluids used for RBC count?

Q.5 Which physiological condition causes a decrease in RBC count?

Decreased count is seen during pregnancy and is due to hemodilution. Increased estrogens and aldosterone cause fluid retention and thus an increase in plasma volume. (The blood volume may increase by about 25% above normal just before term. The red cell mass also increases.

Q.6 Define Anemia, Polycythemia. What are the causes and types?

Experiment No. 13

Aim: Determination of Bleeding time (B. T.)

***Key words*:** Bleeding time, Hemostasis, Platelet plug formation, Bleeding disorders, Methods for bleeding time

INTRODUCTION

The term hemostasis (Greek Hema = blood; stasis= halt) refers to the process of stoppage of bleeding after blood vessels are punctured, cut, or otherwise damaged. Hemostasis, which is a homeostatic mechanism to prevent loss of blood, is a result of a complex, natural, physiological response. The term is also used for surgical arrest of bleeding.

Thus, hemostasis has a high degree of survival value,

Hemostasis involves the following 4 interrelated steps

1. *Vasoconstriction (contraction of injured blood vessels).*
2. *Platelet plug formation.*
   a. Platelet activation
   b. Platelet adhesion
   c. platelet release reaction
   d. platelet aggregation
3. *Formation of a blood clot.*
4. *Fibrinolysis (dissolution of the clot).*

The bleeding time test is a useful tool to test for platelet plug formation and capillary integrity. Therefore BT test is considered as *in vitro* test of platelet function. Occasionally, the bleeding time test will be ordered on a patient scheduled for surgery. The bleeding time is dependent upon the efficiency of tissue fluid in accelerating the coagulation process, on capillary function and the number of blood platelets present and their ability to form a platelet plug. Prolonged bleeding times are generally found when the platelet count is below 50,000/μL, and when there is platelet dysfunction. When a patient is suspected of having a bleeding disorder, several tests are performed to screen defect(s) of primary hemostasis. These tests include the bleeding time, prothrombin time, activated partial thromboplastin time and platelet count.

Formation of the Platelet Plug

If the cut in the blood vessel is very small, the cut is often sealed by a *platelet plug,* rather than by a blood clot. To understand this, it is important that we first discuss the nature of platelets themselves.

Physical and Chemical Characteristics of Platelets

Platelets also called *thrombocytes* are minute discs 1 to 4 micrometres in diameter. They are formed in the bone marrow from *megakaryocytes*, which are extremely large cells of the hematopoietic series in the marrow; the megakaryocytes fragment into the minute platelets either in the bone marrow or soon after entering the blood, especially as they squeeze through capillaries.

The normal concentration of platelets in the blood is between 150,000 and 300,000 per microlitre of blood.

Platelets have many functional characteristics of whole cells, even though they do not have nuclei and cannot reproduce.

Cytoplasm of platelets is filled with several active factors such as:

(1) *Actin* and *myosin molecules*, which are contractile proteins similar to those found in muscle cells,

and still another contractile protein, *thrombosthenin*, that can cause the platelets to contract.

(2) Residuals of both the *endoplasmic reticulum* and the *Golgi apparatus* that synthesize various enzymes and especially store large quantities of calcium ions.

(3) Mitochondria and enzyme systems capable of forming *adenosine triphosphate* (ATP) and *adenosine diphosphate* (ADP).

(4) Enzyme systems that synthesize *prostaglandins*, which are local hormones that cause many vascular and other local tissue reactions.

(5) F*ibrin-stabilizing factor*, an important protein which plays key role in to blood coagulation.

(6) *A growth factor* that causes vascular endothelial cells, vascular smooth muscle cells, and fibroblasts to multiply and grow, thus causing cellular growth that eventually helps repair damaged vascular walls.

The cell membrane of the platelets is also important. On its surface is a coat of *glycoproteins* that repulses adherence to normal endothelium and yet causes adherence to *injured* areas of the vessel wall, especially to injured endothelial cells and even more so to any exposed collagen from deep within the vessel wall. In addition, the platelet membrane contains large amounts of *phospholipids* that activate multiple stages in the blood-clotting process.

Mechanism of the Platelet Plug

When platelets come in contact with a damaged vascular surface, especially with collagen fibers in the vascular wall, the platelets themselves immediately change their own characteristics drastically. They begin to swell; they assume irregular forms with numerous irradiating pseudopods protruding from their surfaces; their contractile proteins contract forcefully and cause the release of granules that contain multiple active factors; they become sticky so that they adhere to collagen in the tissues and to a protein called *von Willebrand factor* that leaks into the traumatized tissue from the plasma; they secrete large quantities of ADP; and their enzymes form *thromboxane* A_2. The ADP and thromboxane in turn act on nearby platelets to activate them as well, and the stickiness of these additional platelets causes them to adhere to the original activated platelets. Therefore, at the site of any opening in a blood vessel wall, the damaged vascular wall activates successively increasing numbers of platelets that themselves attract more and more additional platelets, thus forming a *platelet plug*. This is at first a loose plug, but it is usually successful in blocking blood loss if the vascular opening is small. Then, during the subsequent process of blood coagulation, *fibrin threads* form. These attach tightly to the platelets, thus constructing an unyielding plug (Fig. 13.1).

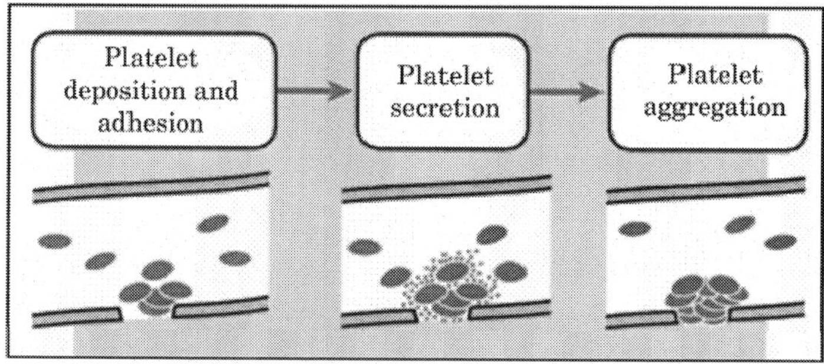

Fig. 13.1: Mechanism of the Platelet Plug

Importance of the Platelet Plug

The platelet-plugging mechanism is extremely important for closing minute ruptures in very small blood vessels that occur many thousands of times daily. Indeed, multiple small holes through the endothelial cells themselves are often closed by platelets actually fusing with the endothelial cells to form additional endothelial cell membrane. A person who has few blood platelets develops each day literally thousands of small hemorrhagic areas under the skin and throughout the internal tissues, but this does not occur in the normal person.

Physiological Basis of Bleeding Disorders

Bleeding disorders may be inherited or acquired—the acquired defects being more common. Disorders due to platelet and vessel wall defects are more common than coagulation disorders that are due to deficiencies of clotting factors.

Excessive and prolonged bleeding with small injuries, or spontaneous bleeding may result from defects of:

A. Platelets
B. Blood vessel walls
C. Coagulation of blood.

Defects of Platelets and Vessel Walls

Defects of platelets and vessel walls typically cause spontaneous bleeding from small vessels, or during cuts and bruises (*e.g.* pinpoint hemorrhages and purpuric lesions in the skin (blue-red patches), and bleeding in the gums.

DEFINITION

Bleeding Time

Bleeding Time (BT) is the time interval between the skin puncture and spontaneous, unassisted cessation of bleeding.

Four procedures are currently in use for determining the bleeding time: the Duke method, the Ivy Method, the Mielke Method and the Simplate or Surgicutt Methods.

Duke Method

1. A standardized puncture of the fingertip/ear lobe is made, and the length of time required for bleeding to cease while the blood is being blotted every 30 seconds is recorded.
2. A lancet is used to make the puncture.
3. No repeat testing is allowed due to space.

4. Causes apprehension in the patient.
5. This test method is the easiest to perform, but is the least standardized and has the worst precision and accuracy.
6. Normal value: 1 -5 min.

Ivy Method

1. A blood pressure cuff is used to maintain constant pressure within the capillaries to help standardize the procedure. The cuff is inflated to 40 mm Hg on the upper arm to control capillary tone and to improve the sensitivity and reproducibility.
2. The forearm is the bleeding time site used.
3. A sterile, disposable blood lancet is used and the length of time required for bleeding to cease is recorded.
4. The greatest source of variation in this test is largely due to difficulty in performing a standardized puncture. This usually leads to erroneously low results.
5. *Normal value*: up to 9 min.

Mielke Method

1. Modification of the Ivy Method.
2. A Bard-Parker or similar disposable blade is used, along with a rectangular polystyrene or plastic template that contains a standardized slit. The blade is placed in a special handle containing a gauge in order to standardize the depth of the incision.
3. The same procedure as described for the Surgicutt method is employed.
4. Advantages of this method include:
   a. That the surgical incision more closely approximates the patient's hemostatic response to surgery, when compared to the puncture in the Ivy Method.
   b. The depth of the incision can be controlled.

5. Disadvantages of this method include:
   a. Cost- scalpel and template required sterilization after each use.
   b. Patient apprehension, due to unconcealed scalpel.
   c. Small scars might form.

Simplate/Surgicutt Method: Preferred Method

1. Modification of the Ivy Method.
2. The first bleeding time device introduced was the Simplate. The Simplate device has a trigger and spring method for the blade. The blade has a depth of 1.0 mm and a width of 5.0 mm. Another brand name is the Surgicutt.
3. *Normal bleeding time* = < 7 minutes.
4. Advantages of this method include:
   a. Instrument is a sterile, standardized, easy to use device that makes a uniform incision.
   b. Instrument is a spring activated surgical steel blade which is housed in a plastic unit. This eliminates variability of blade incision.
   c. This method is the most standardized method of all the bleeding time procedures.
   d. Inexpensive
5. Disadvantages of this method include:
   a. Slight scarring can occur so patient should be informed.

Duke's Method

This is the preferred method to be performed at laboratory level with ease. The bleeding site selected may be fingertip. Since the skin of the fingertip is quite thick in some persons, a small cut in the skin of the earlobe with the corner edge of a sterile blade gives better results. The earlobe method is the original "Duke" method for BT.

Principle

A deep skin puncture is made and the time required for bleeding to stop is recorded. The method determines the function of platelets and capillary integrity.

Normal bleeding time = 1–5 minutes.

Materials: Equipment for sterile finger-prick, clean filter papers, Stopwatch.

Chemicals: 70% alcohol or Spirit

Procedure

1. Keep ready filter paper. (With patient name (your own name). Age, Gender, date of test, Name of test, Method) in corner of it. Neatly bordered.
2. Wash the hands properly and allow to dry them.
3. Apply 70 % v/v alcohol with cotton swab to the ball of finger to be pricked (Preferably left hand ring finger.) Allow to dry.
4. Take a bold prick to have deep skin puncture about 3-5 mm depth and immediately start the stop watch.
5. Blot drop of blood from prick on filter paper serially in a row. After every 30 seconds, with the help of stop-watch.
6. Till there is no stain on filter paper *i.e.* when bleeding stops, stop the stop watch.
7. Count and number the spots of blood on filter paper.
8. Calculate and record bleeding time.
9. Compare the result with normal bleeding time (1 to 3 min.)
10. Submit patient report with attached filter paper of blood drops. (Bleeding time is less than clotting time)

Precautions

1. The skin site chosen for BT should be scrubbed well with alcohol to increase the blood flow.
2. The skin should be dry and the puncture should be 3–4 mm deep to give free-flowing blood. Do not squeeze.

3. Do not press the filter paper on the puncture site.
4. If bleeding continues for more than 10–12 minutes, stop the test and press a sterile gauze on the wound. Inform your teacher about the bleeding.

Observations

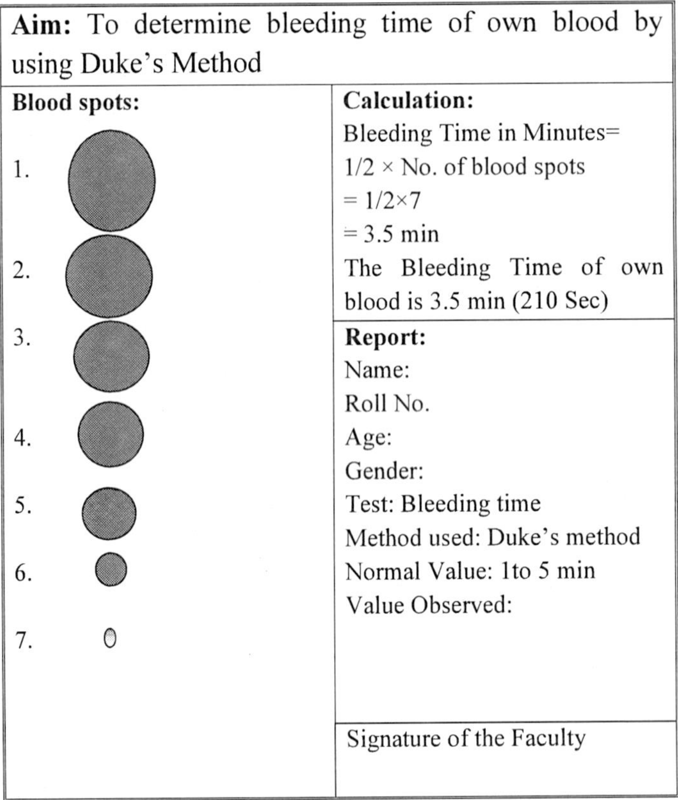

Aim: To determine bleeding time of own blood by using Duke's Method	
Blood spots: 1. 2. 3. 4. 5. 6. 7.	**Calculation:** Bleeding Time in Minutes= 1/2 × No. of blood spots = 1/2×7 = 3.5 min The Bleeding Time of own blood is 3.5 min (210 Sec)
	Report: Name: Roll No. Age: Gender: Test: Bleeding time Method used: Duke's method Normal Value: 1to 5 min Value Observed:
	Signature of the Faculty

***Result*:** The Bleeding time of own blood is .... (Normal bleeding time is 1 to 5 min).

Experiment No. 14

Aim: To Study Blood Coagulation time

***Key words*:** Blood coagulation, Clotting factors, Methods of clotting time, Disorders

BLOOD COAGULATION TIME

Clotting time is the time interval between onset of bleeding and appearance of semisolid mass of blood. It is the time required for a sample of blood to clot or coagulate *in vitro* under standard conditions.

Blood coagulation or clotting is the formation of a jelly like substance over the valves of the blood vessels resulting in stoppage of blood flow. Clotting is a natural defense mechanism to prevent blood loss from the body. Whenever a great blood vessel ruptures, bleeding continues for few minutes. As there is a rush of platelets, a cut or injury is plugged causing to bleeding stops. Thereafter, blood loses its fluidity and sets into a semisolid mass. This mass is referred as clot and the phenomenon is called as blood coagulation. This blood clot is formed by a network of insoluble fibrin fibers in which the formed elements of blood are trapped (Fig. 14.1).

The clot begins to develop in 15 to 20 seconds if the trauma to the vascular wall has been severe, and in 1 to 2 minutes if the trauma has been minor. Activator substances from the traumatized vascular wall, from platelets, and from blood proteins adhering to the traumatized vascular wall initiate the clotting process.

This process of formation of fibrin network or clot is an enzymatic cascade which involves several substances like Ca^{2+}

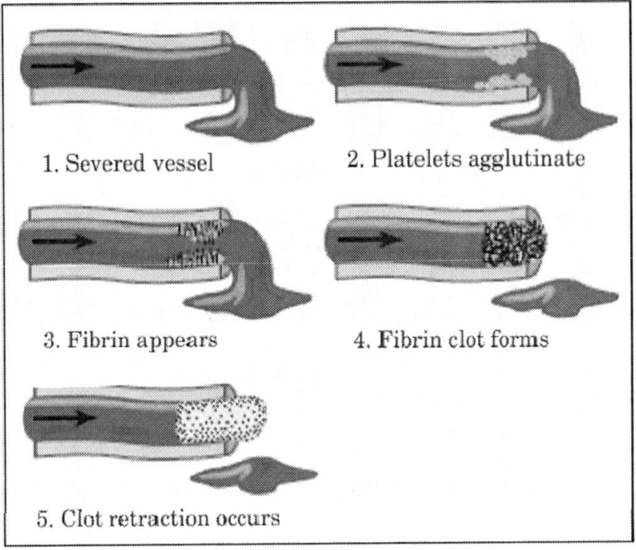

Fig. 14.1: Process of clotting in injured blood vessel

ions, inactive enzymes synthesized by hepatocytes are called as clotting factors. Most clotting factors are identified by roman numerical that indicate their order of discovery (Table 14.1).

Clotting is initiated by two pathways *i.e.* intrinsic pathway and extrinsic pathway. (Fig. 14.2, Fig. 14.3, Fig. 14.4).

Defects of Clotting

Defects of clotting are of 2 types:

(a) ***Excessive bleeding into tissues*** (muscles, joints, viscera, etc.) is usually due to injury to relatively large vessels. The delay in the formation of a clot fails to support the normal action of platelets in checking blood loss. Deficiency of clotting factors—inherited or in liver disease (hepatitis, cirrhosis and vitamin K deficiency) are the usual causes.

(b) ***Thrombosis*:** It is clotting of blood that occurs within unbroken blood vessels. A roughened endothelium due to arteriosclerosis, infection, or injury is the common cause.

Table14.1: Clotting Factors in Blood with Synonyms, source and pathways of activation

Number	*Name/s*	*Source*	*Pathways of activation*
I	Fibrinogen	Liver	Common
II	Prothrombin	Liver	Common
III	Tissue thromboplastin (TPL) (tissue factor, (TF)	Damaged tissues and activated platelets	Extrinsic
IV	Calcium ions (Ca^{2+})	Diet, bones, platelets	All
V	Proaccelerin (accelerator-factor)	Liver and platelets globulin, AcG; labile	Extrinsic and intrinsic
VI	There is no such factor.	—	—
VII	Proconvertin; stable factor; serum pro-thrombin conversion accelerator (SPCA)	Liver	Extrinsic
VIII	Antihemophilic factor (AHF); antihemophilic factor A; antihemophilic globulin (AHG)	Platelets and endothelial cells	Intrinsic
IX	Christmas factor (CF); antihemophilic factor B (AHF-B) plasma thromboplastin component (PTC)	Liver	Intrinsic
X	Stuart factor, Prower factor Stuart-Prower factor; thrombokinase	Liver	Extrinsic and Intrinsic
XI	Plasma thromboplastin antecedent; antihemophilic factor C	Liver	Intrinsic
XII	Hageman factor; glass contact factor; glass factor; contact factor;	Liver	Intrinsic
XIII	Fibrin stabilizing factor (FSF); Laki-Lorand factor	Liver and platelets	Common

Methods for Clotting Time Determination

CT is Susually determined by two methods

1. Capillary tube method
2. Lee-White method

   Capillary tube method is routinely used for CT determination in clinical laboratories

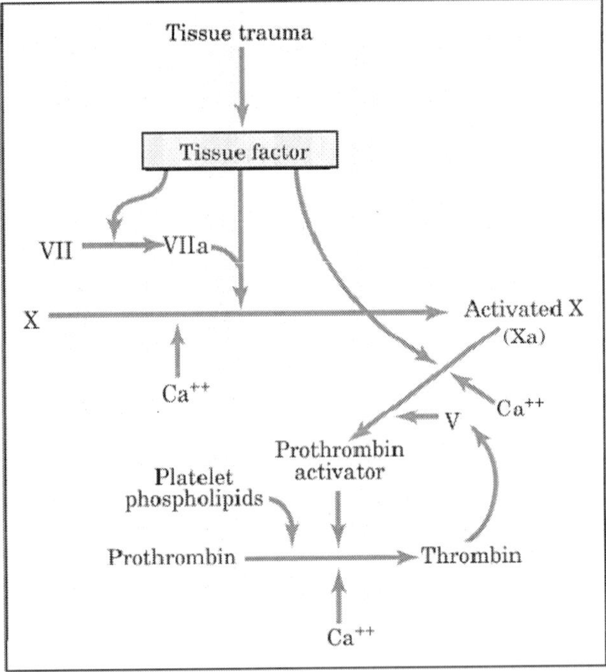

Fig. 14.2: Extrinsic pathway of blood coagulation

Capillary Tube Method

Principle

A standard incision is made in the skin of the patient and the blood is taken into a capillary glass tube. The length of time that it takes for the blood to clot is reported. Clotting is confirmed by the appearance of fibrin string is reported as CT.

Apparatus and Chemicals

Materials for sterile finger prick, capillary tube (10-15 cm in length and 1-1.5 mm in diameter), Stopwatch, cotton swabs, 70% alcohol or spirit.

Procedure

1. Sterile the finger tip with cotton swab soaked in 70% alcohol. Allow it to dry naturally.

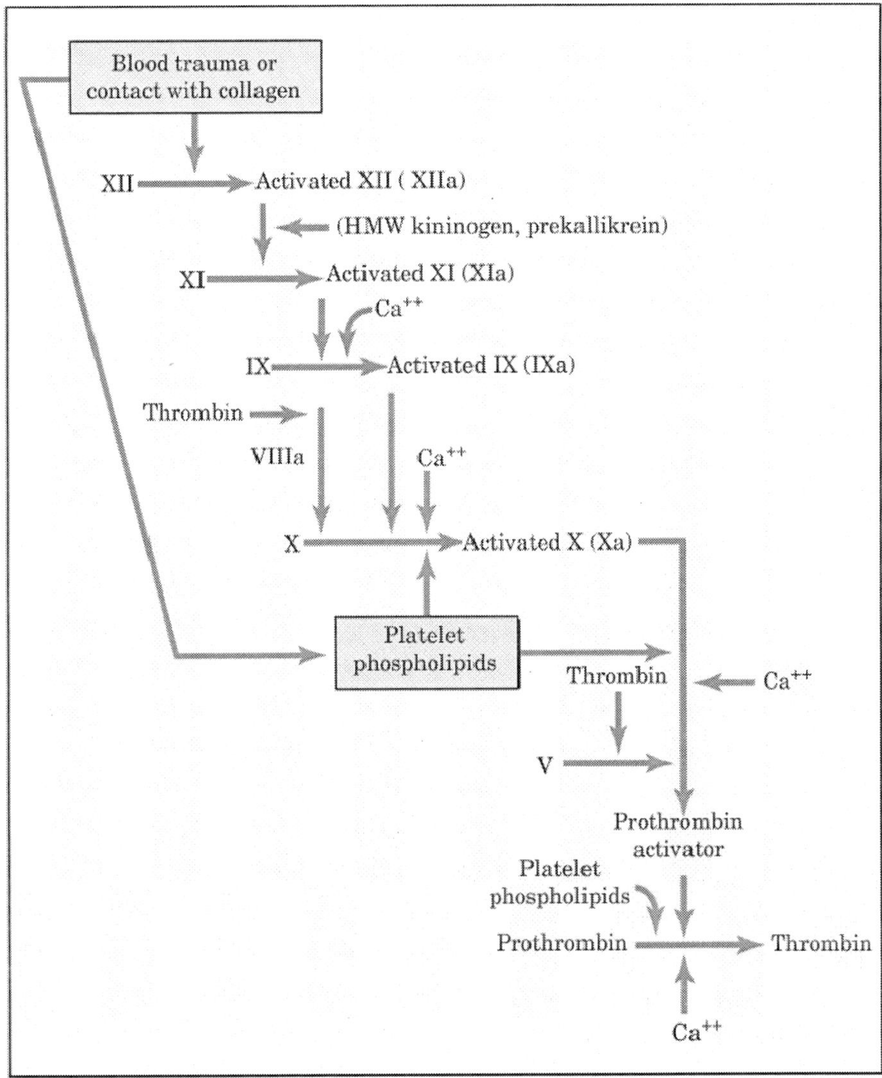

Fig. 14.3: Intrinsic pathway of blood coagulation

2. Make a bold finger prick (3 mm deep) with usual aseptic precautions. Immediately start the stop watch as soon as blood is visible.
3. Wipe the first drop of blood and allow the next drop of blood to form.

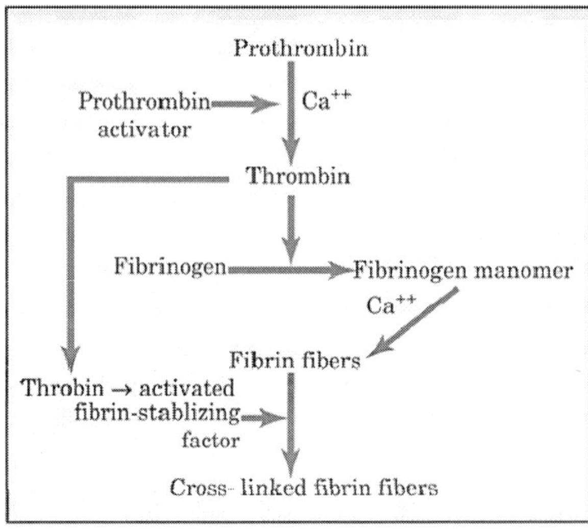

Fig. 14.4: Common pathway of blood coagulation

4. Dip one end of the capillary into blood drop gently without pressure and allow the blood to flow into the capillary. While doing this, hold the other end of capillary at lower level.
5. Allow to fill the capillary with blood by lowering the end of fitted capillary around ¾th of its length.
6. Hold the capillary tube between the palms of your hands to keep the blood near body temperature.
7. After 2 minutes, break off 1 cm bits of glass tube from one end, at intervals of 30 seconds, and look for the formation of fibrin threads between the broken ends. (Fig. 14.5)
8. The end-point is reached when fibrin threads span a gap of 5 mm between the broken ends.

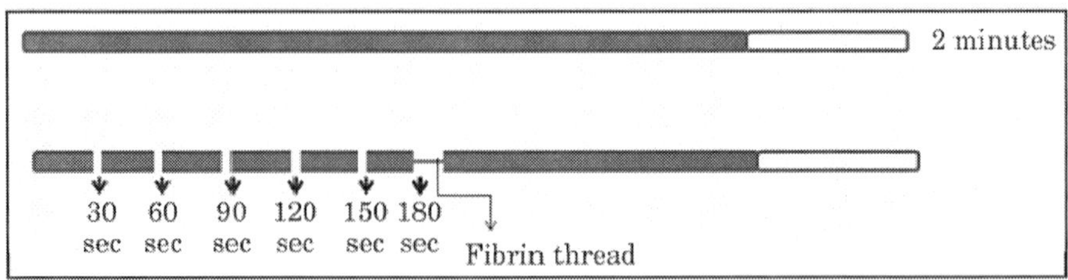

Fig. 14.5: Breaking the capillary and formation of fibrin thread

9. Repeat breaking at regular time intervals, till fibrin thread appears at the broken end of capillary tube. Do not pull away the cut pieces ling apart and bristly.
10. The end-point is reached when fibrin threads span a gap of 5 mm between the broken ends.
11. Record time interval between pricking finger and first appearance of fibrin thread at the broken ends of capillary tube. That is clotting time of blood.

    Normal clotting time by capillary glass method = 2–8 minutes.

Precautions

1. Prick should be bold enough to allow free flow of blood
2. Capillary should be held in between palms immediately after filling to maintain temperature. As temperature affects clotting.
3. Appearance of fibrin thread should be observed at each break.

Observations

RESULT

The Clotting time of own blood is .... (Normal clotting time is 2 to 8 min).

DISCUSSION

The clotting of blood with this method involves both the intrinsic and the extrinsic systems of clotting. There is injury to the blood (coming in contact with glass, intrinsic pathway), and the injury to the tissues (extrinsic pathway).

The CT is prolonged in hemophilia and other clotting disorders, because thrombin cannot normally be generated. Yet, the BT, which reflects platelet plug formation and vasoconstriction, independently of clot formation, is normal.

Clotting factor deficiencies may prolong clotting time. If CT is more than 10 minutes, detailed investigation should be carried out to identify the missing factors.

QUESTIONS

Q.1 What is the clinical importance of doing BT and CT?

BT and CT are important in the following situations:

i. History of frequent and persistent bleeding from minor injuries, or spontaneous bleeding into tissues.
ii. Before every minor and major surgery (tooth extraction, etc.).
iii. Before taking biopsy, especially from bone marrow, liver, kidney, etc.
iv. Before and during anticoagulant therapy.
v. Family history of bleeding disorders.

Q.2 How does BT differ from CT? What is the interrelation between them, and which aspects of hemostasis are tested by them?

Both BT and CT are done together in all disorders of hemostasis. They are interrelated in the sense that platelets are involved in both tests. The BT tests the platelet plug formation and the *condition of the microvessels (arterioles, capillaries, venules), while CT tests the formation of the clot.* Increase in BT (*e.g.* in purpura), or CT (*e.g.* in hemophilia) usually occur independently of each other.

Q.3 What are the factors on which BT and CT depend?

Bleeding time depends on

i. Breadth and depth of the wound.
ii. Degree of hyperemia of the skin puncture site.
iii. Number of platelets and their functional status.
iv. Functional status of the blood vessels.
v. Temperature: In cold weather, low temperature promotes vasoconstriction and thus shortens BT.

Clotting time depends on

i. Nature of contact surface (glass in this case; siliconized surface would prolong the CT.

ii. Presence or absence of clotting factors.
iii. Temperature: Low temperature may prolong the CT.

Q.4 Name the conditions in which only the bleeding time is prolonged while the clotting time is normal.

Pronged BT, with normal CT is seen in the following conditions:

A. ***Low Platelet Count (Thrombocytopenia)*:** It may be due to:

i. Decreased production of platelets
ii. Increased destruction of platelets.

B. ***Functional Platelet Defects*:** Prolonged BT with normal platelet count suggests the following defects:

i. ***Drugs*:** aspirin, large doses of penicillin, other drugs.
ii. ***Von Willebrand disease*:** Inherited as an autosomal dominant trait, this condition is associated with a deficiency of a component of factor VIII called "factor VIII related antigen (VIII R: Ag; vWF) which acts as a carrier of factor VIII
iii. ***Other diseases*:** uremia, cirrhosis, leukemia, etc.

C. ***Vessel wall defects*:** These defects are generally acquired, but may be inherited.

i. ***Prolonged treatment with corticosteroids*:** Also other drugs penicillin, sulphas, and aspirin, etc. may damage vessel walls. There may be severe bleeding in a known case of purpura if aspirin is inadvertently administered.
ii. ***Allergic purpura*:** There is damage to capillary walls by antibodies.
iii. ***Infections:*** Infections such as typhus, bacterial endocarditis, hemolytic streptococci.
iv. ***Deficiency of vitamin C:*** Petechia, and bleeding from gums occur due to decreased intercellular substance and less stable capillary basement membrane.
v. ***Senile purpura*:** In the elderly, purpuric hemorrhages occur on the back of the hands and forearms due to prolonged pressure or mild trauma. Small vessels rupture due to increased mobility of skin resulting from loss of elastic and connective tissues around blood vessels.

vi. ***Connective tissue diseases*:** Some of these diseases may be associated with purpuric bleeding.

Q.5. Name the conditions where the clotting time is increased and those where it is decreased.

The coagulation time is increased in the following conditions:

A. ***Hereditary Coagulation Disorders*:**

1. *Hemophilias*—A, B, C, D
2. ***Von Willebrand disease*:** Though usually a bleeding disease, variant forms show reduced factor VIII activity and an increase in CT. Acquired forms are caused by antibodies which inhibit vWF. The laboratory and clinical features are similar to hemophilia A.
3. ***A fibrinogenemia and dysfibrinogenemia*:** The concentration of fibrinogen may be greatly reduced (normal = 250 to 300 mg%) or absent or it may be chemically abnormal, though both may be present at the same time.
4. *Deficiency of factor XIII and defective cross-linking* is a rare disorder.

B. Acquired Coagulation Disorders: These may develop in a variety of diseases as mentioned below:

1. ***Vitamin K deficiency***: Deficiency of vitamin K (major sources: green vegetables, also gut bacteria) may be due to inadequate intake, intestinal malabsorption (obstructive jaundice), or loss of storage sites in liver. Since it acts a cofactor in the synthesis of prothrombin, and factors VII, IX and X, its deficiency leads to fall in their levels.
2. *Liver diseases*: There is a decrease of all clotting factors except VIII. There is also a reduced uptake of vitamin K, and abnormalities of platelet function.
3. *Intravascular clotting:* Clotting factors are used up and bleeding may occur.
4. *Anticoagulant therapy:* Patients receiving heparin or warfarin show an increased CT.

C. *Newborns:* Newborns, especially premature babies sometimes have a tendency to bleed because the plasma levels of certain factors are low, especially prothrombin. Usually, these levels reach normal by the 2nd or 3rd week after birth. Vitamin K is given if bleeding persists.

The Clotting Time is decreased in

***Physiological conditions*:** malnutrition, parturition.

***Pathological conditions*:** There is no pathological condition in which the CT is decreased.

Experiment No. 15

Aim: To Study Estimation of hemoglobin content

***Key words*:** Hemoglobin, Structure, Types, Different methods of estimation, Sahli's acid

INTRODUCTION

Hemoglobin (also spelled haemoglobin and abbreviated Hb or Hgb) is the iron-containing oxygen-transport metalloprotein in the red blood cells of vertebrates, and the tissues of some invertebrates.

A substance contained within erythrocytes (red blood cells) that is responsible for their color and their remarkably high oxygen-carrying capacity. Hemoglobin is the most efficient oxygen-carrier known. Oxyhemoglobin is scarlet in color; reduced hemoglobin is of a purplish color.

In mammals, the protein makes up about 97% of the red blood cells dry content, and around 35% of the total content (including water).

Hemoglobin transports oxygen from the lungs or gills to the rest of the body (*i.e.* the tissues) where it releases the oxygen for cell use.

Hemoglobin is also found in outside red blood cells and their progenitor lines. Other cells that contain hemoglobin include the A9 dopaminergic neurons in the substantia nigra, macrophages, alveolar cells, and mesangial cells in the kidney. In these tissues, hemoglobin has a non-oxygen carrying function as an antioxidant and a regulator of iron metabolism.

In most humans, the hemoglobin molecule is an assembly of four globular protein subunits. Each subunit is composed of a protein chain tightly associated with a non-protein heme group. Each protein chain arranges into a set of alpha-helix structural segments connected together in a globin fold arrangement, so called because this arrangement is the same folding motif used in other heme/ globin proteins such as myoglobin. This folding pattern contains a pocket which strongly binds the heme group.

Myoglobin is an oxygen-binding protein found in the muscle tissue of vertebrates in general and in almost all mammals.

Myoglobin (abbreviated Mb) is a single-chain globular protein of 153 or 154 amino acids, containing a haem (iron-containing porphyrin) prosthetic group in the center around which the remaining apoprotein folds.

The normal hemoglobin content in human varies with altitude. Normal hemoglobin content for male is in the range of 13.8 to 17.2 g/dL, while female falls in the range of 12.1 to 15.1 g/dL.

Structure of Haemoglobin

Haemoglobin is a large protein molecule folded around four iron atoms and it has a quaternary structure. A quaternary structure is where two or more polypeptide chains join together due to chemical bonds which could be ionic, covalent or hydrogen bonds. (Fig. 15.1).

In the case of haemoglobin there are four polypeptide chains. Each one of these polypeptide chains contains a haem group which is able to bind to one oxygen molecule. Therefore four oxygen molecules can be transported by each haemoglobin molecule. In every red blood cell there are approximately 270 million haemoglobin molecules and so each red blood cell can carry about 1080 million oxygen molecules!

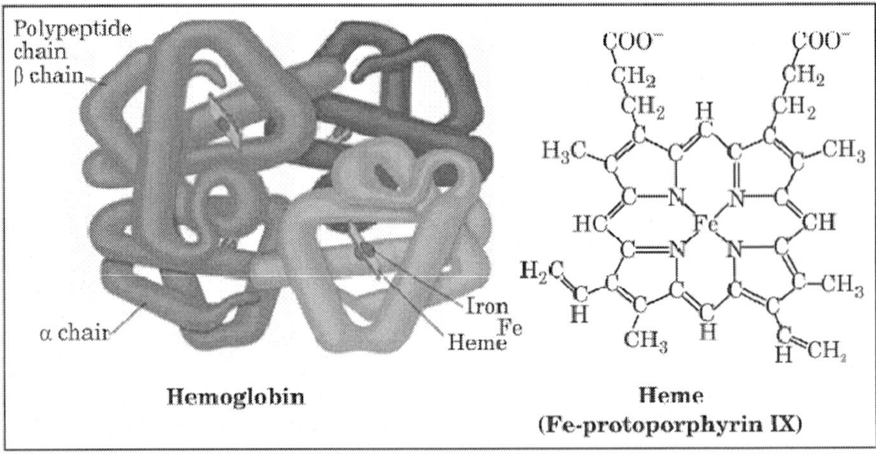

Fig. 15.1: Structure of haemoglobin

Types of Haemoglobin

There are seven types of haemoglobin molecules throughout a human's life. Four when you are an embryo, one once you develop into a fetus and then as an adult you have two.

Embryonic Haemoglobin

The form of haemoglobin most common and in highest proportion in an embryo is Haemoglobin Gower I ($\zeta_2\varepsilon_2$) The four polypeptide chains that compose this type of haemoglobin are two zeta and two epsilon chains.

The other three forms of haemoglobin are present at much lower levels and are:

- Haemoglobin Gower II ($\alpha_2\varepsilon_2$) – Composed of two alpha and two epsilon chains.
- Haemoglobin Portland I ($\zeta_2\gamma_2$) – Comprised of two zeta and two gamma polypeptides.
- Haemoglobin Portland II ($\zeta_2\beta_2$) – Made of two zeta and two beta polypeptide chains.

Fetal Haemoglobin

Once an embryo develops into a fetus and the four types of embryonic haemoglobin molecules disappear they are replaced by Haemoglobin F($\alpha_2\gamma_2$).

This type of haemoglobin is used due to it having a greater affinity for oxygen than adult haemoglobin. Therefore the growing fetus is able to take its mother's oxygen which is in her bloodstream.

Adult haemoglobin

Haemoglobin F remains in the child's blood until it is around six months old and then almost all of it is replaced with adult haemoglobin.

The two types of adult Haemoglobin are:

- Haemoglobin A ($\alpha_2\beta_2$) – Has two alpha chains and two beta chains
- Haemoglobin A_2 ($\alpha_2\delta_2$) – Has two alpha polypeptides and two delta polypeptides.

There is also a small amount of Haemoglobin F remaining.

Haemoglobin A is the most prevalent as it makes up about 97% of adult haemoglobin.

Variant Forms

As with all biological substances mutations can occur and these mutations cause a change in the genes coding for haemoglobin and so variant forms of haemoglobin are formed. There are several hundred variant forms of haemoglobin.

Thankfully, most variant forms of haemoglobin cause little to no problems. However, there are a select few that do; most notably Haemoglobin S.

Haemoglobin S has a slight change in the coding for the beta chain in adult haemoglobin and this causes sickle cell anaemia.

METHODS

The different methods of estimation of haemoglobin can be classified in to the following categories:

A. Visual methods
   1. Sahli's method
   2. Dare's method
   3. Haden's method
   4. Wintrobe's method
   5. Haldane's method
   6. Tallquist's method

B. Gasometric method

C. Spectrophotometric method
   1. Oxyhaemoglobin method
   2. Cyanmethaemoglobin method

D. Automated hemoglobinometry

E. Other methods
   1. Alkaline hematin method
   2. Specific gravity method
   3. Comparator method.

SAHLI'S ACID HEMATIN METHOD

Principle

Anticoagulated blood is added to the 0.1 N HCl and kept for 5-7 minutes to form acid haematin. The color of this acid haematin should be matched with the solution, present in the calibration tube. Distilled water is added to the acid haematin until the color matches and the final reading is directly noted from the graduation in the calibration tube.

Requirements

1. Sahli's hemoglobinometer

   Sahli's graduated hemoglobin tube (marked in grams percent G % (2-24) and percentage % (10-140) (Fig. 15.2).

   Comparator with a brown glass standard. Opaque white glass is present at the back to provide uniform illumination.

   Sahli's pipette or hemoglobin pipette (marked at 20 μl or 0.02 ml). No bulb

   Stirrer: Thin glass rod.
2. N/10 HCL
3. Distilled water
4. Dropper
5. Materials for a sterile finger prick

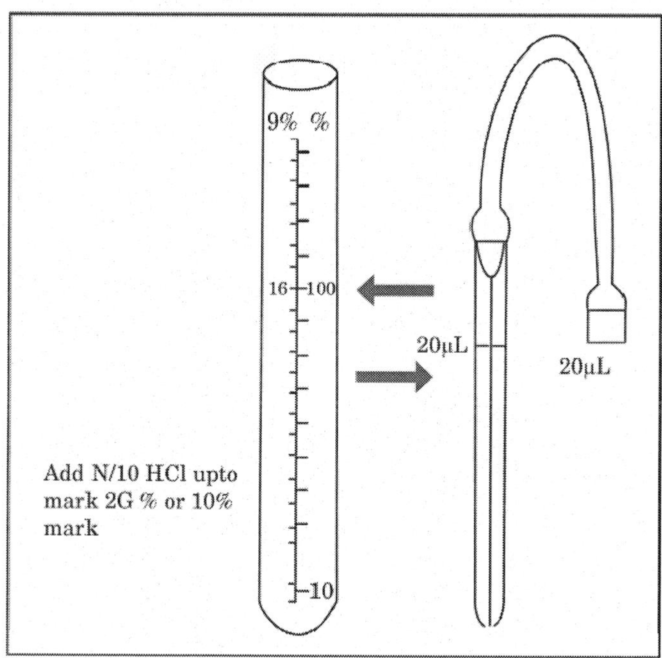

Fig. 15.2: Sahli's graduated hemoglobin tube and pipette

Procedure

1. After ensuring the hemoglobin pipette and tube are dry, add N/10 HCl into the tube upto mark 2G% or 10% in to graduated tube.
2. Fill the pipette with blood up to 20 μL mark. Make sure that no air bubbles enter into the pipette. If it enters, discard and pipette again. Wipe the external surface of the pipette to remove any excess blood.
3. Add the blood into the tube containing N/10 HCl. Wash out the contents of the hemoglobin pipette by drawing in and blowing out the acid few times so that the blood is mixed with the acid thoroughly.
4. Allow to stand undisturbed for 10 min. (This is because, maximum conversion of hemoglobin to acid hematin, occurs in the first ten minutes).
5. Place the hemoglobinometer tube in the comparator and add distilled water to the solution drop by drop. Stir with the glass rod till its color matches with that of the comparator glass. While matching the color, the glass rod must be removed from the solution and held vertically in the tube. (Note that the stirrer should be above the level of the solution and not out of the tube) (Fig. 15.3).
6. The reading of the lower meniscus of the solution should be noted as the result.
7. Express the hemoglobin content as G %.

Precautions

I. Pipetting of blood should be done cautiously
II. Mix the blood properly with HCl by using stirrer
III. Match the color cautious; Fig. 15.3: Sahli's hemoglobinometer

OBSERVATIONS AND RESULTS

Compare your color matching with that of your work-partner and record the observations in your workbook. Take the average of 3

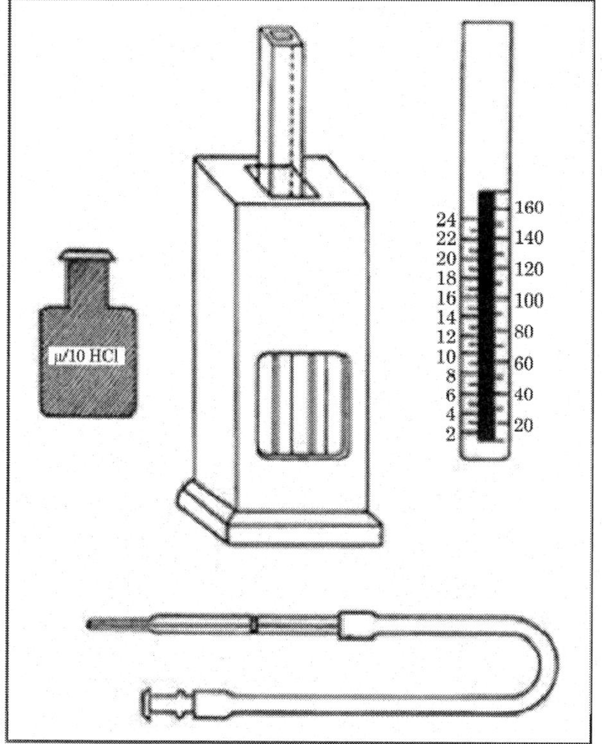

Fig. 15.3: Sahli's hemoglobinometer

readings as shown below, and report your result as: Hb = ...g/dl.

- *1st reading*, when the color is slightly darker than the standard: ....g/dl.
- *2nd reading,* when, after adding a few drops of distilled water, the color exactly matches the standard: .... g/dl.
- *3rd reading,* when, after adding some more drops, the color becomes a little lighter than the standard:................... g/dl.

  For report. Express your result as: Hb= ....g/dl.
- ***Oxygen carrying capacity*:** Knowing your Hb concentration, and that 1.0 g of Hb can carry 1.34 ml of O_2, calculate its oxygen-carrying capacity as ....ml O_2/dl.

- ***Color index (CI)*:** This is the ratio of Hb% and RBC%

  CI = Hb%/ RBC%

  100% Hb = 14.8 g/dL

  100% RBC = 5 million/ mm^3

***Normal Values*:** 0.85 to 1.10, values less than 0.85 indicates hypochromic anaemia

Report

Sr. No	*Parameter*	*Obtained Value*
1	Hb G% *Normal Value* In male 13.8 to 17.2 g/dL, In female 12.1 to 15.1 g/dL.	
2	Hb %	
3	Oxygen carrying capacity *Normal Value* 18.5 cc	
4	Percent oxygen carrying capacity	
5	Color index *Normal Value* 0.85-1.10	

Experiment No. 16

Aim: To Determine the Blood Group of Own Blood Sample

***Key words*:** Blood, Transfusion, ABO system, Landsteiner's law, Rh system, Methods for determination

INTRODUCTION

Transfusion of blood is a life-saving procedure in all the condition where there is loss of blood like anemias. On the other hand, blood can only be given after blood grouping which is a necessary condition before blood is administered to any individual. Blood grouping is also done to settle paternity disputes and other medicolegal purposes. The surface of erythrocytes contains a genetically determined assortment of antigens composed of glycoproteins and glycolipids. These are called as agglutinogenes. Based on the presence and absence of antigens, blood is categorized in to two different groups as ABO system and Rh system.

THE ABO SYSTEM

The surface of a red blood cell is coated with a combination of sugars and proteins called antigens. Depending on combination, it will have A antigens, B antigens, no antigens or both A and B antigens. It is the presence of the A and B antigens and corresponding antibodies in the clear part of blood called plasma that determines an individual's blood group.

The most important blood groups in transfusion are the ABO blood group system. The four main blood groups in the ABO system are:

- ***Blood group A*** – has A antigens on the red blood cells with anti-B antibodies in the plasma
- ***Blood group B*** – has B antigens with anti-A antibodies in the plasma
- ***Blood group O*** – has no antigens, but both anti-A and anti-B antibodies in the plasma
- ***Blood group AB*** – has both A and B antigens, but no antibodies

The table below shows the possible permutations of antigens and antibodies with the corresponding ABO type ("yes" indicates the presence of a component and "no" indicates its absence in the blood of an individual).

LANDSTEINER'S LAW

1. "If an agglutinogen is present in the red cells of a blood, the corresponding agglutinin must be absent from the plasma."

2. "If an agglutinogen is absent in the red cells of a blood, the corresponding agglutinin must be present in it's plasma." (Table 16.1).

Table 16.1: Landsteiner's law

ABO Blood Type	*Antigen A*	*Antigen B*	*Antibody Anti- A*	*Antibody Anti- B*
A	Yes	No	No	Yes
B	No	Yes	Yes	No
O	No	No	Yes	Yes
AB	Yes	Yes	No	No

APPLICABILITY

1. The first law is applicable to all groups and types of blood. It is a logical conclusion.
2. The second part is a fact, but not necessarily true always. It is a fact for ABO Blood groups.

3. The Rh, M, N and other groups or types do not follow the second part of the Landsteiner's Law.

The Rh System

Red blood cells sometimes have another antigen, a protein known as the RhD antigen. If this is present, in blood group then it is RhD positive. If it's absent, blood group is RhD negative.

This means it can be one of eight blood groups:

- A RhD positive (A+)
- A RhD negative (A-)
- B RhD positive (B+)
- B RhD negative (B-)
- O RhD positive (O+)
- O RhD negative (O-)
- AB RhD positive (AB+)
- AB RhD negative (AB-)

About 85% of population is RhD positive (36% of the population has O^+, the most common type). In most cases, O RhD negative blood (O^-) can safely be given to anyone. It's often used in medical emergencies when the blood type isn't immediately known. It's safe for most recipients because it doesn't have any A, B or RhD antigens on the surface of the cells, and is compatible with every other ABO and RhD blood group.

Cross Matching

The red cells and the plasma of the donor and recipient blood are separated by centrifugation. The donor red cells are then treated (tested) with the recipient plasma (*major side cross match),* and the donor plasma is tested against the red cells of the recipient (*minor cross match*). The whole process is called "cross matching'. If there is no agglutination in either case, the donor blood can safely be given to the recipient.

Methods for Determination of Blood Groups

1. *Slide Method*

The slide test is relatively the least sensitive method among others for BG determination, but due to its prompt results, it is very much valuable in emergency cases. In this method, a glass slide or white porcelain support is divided into three parts, as for each part, a drop of donor or recipient blood is mixed with anti-A, anti-B and anti-D separately. The agglutination or blood clumping pattern can be visually observed from which the ABO and rhesus D (RhD) type of blood can be determined. The test completes in 5–10 min and is inexpensive, which requires only a small volume of blood typing reagents. However, it is an insensitive method and only useful in preliminary BG matching for getting an early result. The test cannot be conducted for weakly or rarely reactive antigens from which the results are difficult to interpret, and additionally, a low titer of anti-A or anti-B could lead to false positive or false negative results. Although the slide test is useful for outdoor blood typing, it is not reliable enough for completely safe transfusion.

2. *Tube Test*

In comparison to the slide test, the tube test is more sensitive and reliable; therefore, it can be used conveniently for blood transfusion. In this method, both forward (cell), as well as reverse (serum) grouping is carried out. The forward grouping suggests the presence or absence of A and B antigens in RBCs, whereas reverse grouping indicates the presence or absences of anti-A and anti-B in serum. In forward grouping, blood cells are placed in two test tubes along with saline as a diluents media, and then one drop of each anti-A and anti-B is added separately in these samples. These tubes are subjected to centrifugation for few minutes, and then, the resultant matrix is gently shaken for observing agglutination. For precise blood grouping, the two tubes can be categorized according to the extent of blood clumping. The purpose of centrifugation is to ensure enhanced chemical interactions, particularly for weaker antibodies to react, thus leading to agglutination. Some potentiators could also be added to promote the agglutination; moreover, the long incubation of tubes also favors these reactions without drying of the test samples. In a similar fashion, reverse grouping can be performed, as here, the blood serum is treated against RBC reagent groups of A1 and B, and the subsequent agglutination pattern is monitored. The grading of agglutinates in both forward and reverse grouping is useful in comparing the difference in the strength of hemolysis reactions. In general, the tube method is much more sensitive than the slide test and requires a low volume of reagents, and some unexpected antigens can also be detected; therefore, it is a better option for safer transfusions. However, in infants, reverse grouping is somewhat difficult to perform, since they produce insufficient amounts of antibodies to be determined.

3. *Microplate Technology*

Among classical methods, microplate technology is a further step towards more sensitive and fast blood typing analysis with the feasibility of automation. In this technique, both antibodies in blood plasma and antigens on RBCs can be determined. Typical microplates consist of a large number of small tubes that contain a few µL of reagents, which are treated against the blood samples. Following centrifugation and incubation, the subsequent agglutination can be examined by an automatic read out device. The microplate technique was first introduced in early 1950s; however, since then, considerable developments have been made in the design to improve the performance. The foremost advantage of microplate technology is its fast response, low reagent volumes and high throughput analysis. Apart from microplates, gel cards or strips can also be used for blood grouping in modern immunoassay machines.

4. *Column/Gel Centrifugation*

Column agglutination technology or gel centrifugation is a relatively modern approach that has gained substantial interest in ABO blood grouping, as it intends to establish a standard procedure for quantifying cell agglutination. Here, the column is made of small microtubes that contains gel matrix to trap agglutinates. Blood serum or cells are mixed with anti-A, anti-B and anti-D reagents in microtubes under controlled incubation and centrifugation. The gel particles trap the agglutinates, whereas non-agglutinated blood cells are allowed to pass through the column. The analysis time can be reduced by using glass beads in place of gel material, since in this way, faster centrifugation speeds can be achieved, which leads to rapid results. This technology is sensitive, straight-forward and relatively easy to operate for less trained personnel.

PRINCIPLE BEHIND BLOOD TESTS: *BLOOD CLUMPING OR AGGLUTINATION OBSERVATION*

Compatibility between the blood groups of donor and recipient determines the success of a blood transfusion. The ABO and Rh blood groups are looked at while conducting the test. In a diagnostic lab, Monoclonal antibodies are available for A, B and Rh antigen. Monoclonal antibody against Antigen A (also called Anti-A), comes in a small bottles with droppers; the monoclonal suspension being BLUE in colour. Anti-B comes in YELLOW colour. Anti-D (monoclonal antibody against Rh) is colourless. All the colour codes are universal standards. When the monoclonal antibodies are added one by one to wells that contain the test sample (blood from patient), if the RBCs in that particular sample carry the corresponding Antigen, clumps can be observed in the corresponding wells. A drop of blood is left without adding any of the antibodies; it is used as a control in the experiment. The monoclonal antibody bottles should be stored in a refrigerator. It is recommended to tilt the bottle a couple of times before use in order to resuspend the antibodies that have settled at the bottom of the bottle.

APPARATUS AND MATERIALS

1. Magnifying glass or Microscope. •Slides •Glass dropper with a long nozzle. •Sterile blood lancet or needle. •Sterile cotton/ gauze swabs. •Alcohol. •Slides

2. Clean, dry microscope slides. (A special porcelain tile with 12 depressions is available for this purpose and may be used in place of glass slides).
3. ***Anti-A serum:*** [contains monoclonal anti-A antibodies (against human); these antibodies are also called anti-A or alpha (α) agglutinins]. The anti-A serum can also be obtained from a person with blood group B.
4. ***Anti-B serum:*** [contains monoclonal anti-B antibodies (against human); these antibodies are also called anti-B or beta (β) agglutinins]. The anti-B serum can also be obtained from a person with blood group A.
5. ***Anti-D (anti-Rh) serum:*** [Contains monoclonal anti-Rh (D) antibodies (against human). These antibodies are also called anti-D agglutinins.

PROCEDURE

1. Using a glass- marker, name 3 slides, as A, B, and D on the left corner of each slide.
2. Place type A serum on the slide A and B on slide B whereas anti D serum is to be placed on slide D.
3. Sterilize the finger tip and take a bold prick. Place 1 drop of blood on each slide near the drop of antiserum.
4. Mix the blood sample and serum with the help of another slide.
5. Allow it reacts for 5 minutes but not more than 10 minutes because the reaction may not be complete before 5 minutes and drying may occur after 10 minutes both of these factors may yield false results.
6. Observe the slides for agglutination under Magnifying glass or Microscope

PRECAUTIONS

1. The slides should be dry, dust-free and grease-free.
2. Don't uses edges of slide used for mixing blood sample and antiserum

3. Each time different edge of glass slide must be used for mixing blood sample and antiserum otherwise use separate slides
4. Mark the slides with glass marker to avoid confusion
5. Mix antiserum and blood sample properly with constant stirring with the help of glass slide.

OBSERVATIONS AND RESULTS

It is essential that you should be able to distinguish between *"agglutination"* and *"no agglutination"*. The features of each are:

Agglutination

I. If agglutination occurs, it is usually visible to the naked eye. The hemolysed red cells appear as isolated (separate), dark-red masses (clumps) of different sizes and shapes.
II. There is brick-red coloring of the serum by the hemoglobin released from ruptured red cells.
III. Tilting or rocking the slide a few times, or blowing on it does not break or disperse the clumps.
IV. Under 10 X objective, the clumps are visible as dark masses and the outline of the red cells cannot be seen.

No Agglutination

I. In the "control" mixtures, the red cells may form a bunch, or rouleaux. These sedimented red cells give an orange tinge of a suspension of red cells rather than "isolated dark red masses" of ruptured red cells.
II. The red cells will disperse if you gently blow on the slides, or tilt them a few times.

   Confirm all these features of "no agglutination" under the microscope.

Observation Table

Blood group	*Antigen A*	*Antigen B*	*Anti-D*
A RhD positive (A+)	+	–	+
A RhD negative (A-)	+	–	–
B RhD positive (B+)	–	+	+
B RhD negative (B-)	–	+	–
AB RhD positive (AB+)	+	+	+
AB RhD negative (AB-)	+	+	–
O RhD positive (O+)	–	–	+
O RhD negative (O-)	–	–	–

Agglutination = (+), Non Agglutination = (–)

Observation Table for Own Blood Sample

Sr. No	*Antigen*	*Agglutination*
1.	Antigen A	
2.	Antigen B	
3.	Anti- D	

Experiment No. 17

Aim: To Determine Erythrocyte Sedimentation Rate (ESR)

***Key words*:** Erythrocyte Sedimentation rate, Wintrobe's method, Westergren's method

INTRODUCTION

The *erythrocyte sedimentation rate (ESR)* is a common hematological test for nonspecific detection of inflammation that may be caused by infection, some cancers and certain autoimmune diseases. It can be defined as the rate at which Red Blood Cells (RBCs) *sediment in a period of one hour.*

Principle

When anticoagulated blood is allowed to stand in a narrow vertical glass tube, undisturbed for a period of time, the RBCs – under the influence of gravity- settle out from the plasma. The rate at which they settle is measured as the number of millimetres of clear plasma present at the top of the column after one hour (mm/hr). This mechanism involves three stages:

- ***Stage of aggregation*:** It is the initial stage in which piling up of RBCs takes place. The phenomenon is known as Rouleaux formation. It occurs in the first 10-15 minutes.
- ***Stage of sedimentation*:** It is the stage of actual falling of RBCs in which sedimentation occurs at constant rate. This occurs in 30-40 minutes out of 1 hour, depending upon the length of the tube used.

- ***Stage of packing*:** This is the final stage and is also known as stationary phase. In this, there is a slower rate of falling during which packing of sedimented RBCs in column occurs due to overcrowding. It occurs in final 10 minutes in 1 hour

METHOS OF ESR DETERMINATION

There are two main methods to determine ESR:

- Wintrobe's method
- Westergren's method

Each method produces slightly different results. Mosely and Bull (1991) concluded that Wintrobe's method is more sensitive when the ESR is low, whereas, when the ESR is high, the Westergren's method is preferably an indication of patient's clinical state.

Wintrobe's Method

This method uses Wintrobe's tube, a narrow glass tube closed at the lower end only (Fig. 17.1). The Wintrobe's tube has a *length of 11 cm and internal diameter of 2.5 mm*. It contains 0.7–1 ml of blood. The lower 10 cm are in cm and mm. The marking is 0 at the top and 10 at the bottom for ESR. This tube can also be used for PCV. The marking is 10 at the top and 0 at the bottom for PCV.

SPECIMEN REQUIREMENTS

Whole blood collected in EDTA is the only accept able specimen. Specimens must be brought to the laboratory within 4 hours of the blood draw if kept at room temperature. Alternately, whole blood may be refrigerated and brought to the laboratory within 12 hours of the blood draw Clotted or hemolyzed samples are not acceptable.

REQUIREMENTS

- Anticoagulated blood (EDTA, double oxalate)
- Pasteur pipette
- Timer

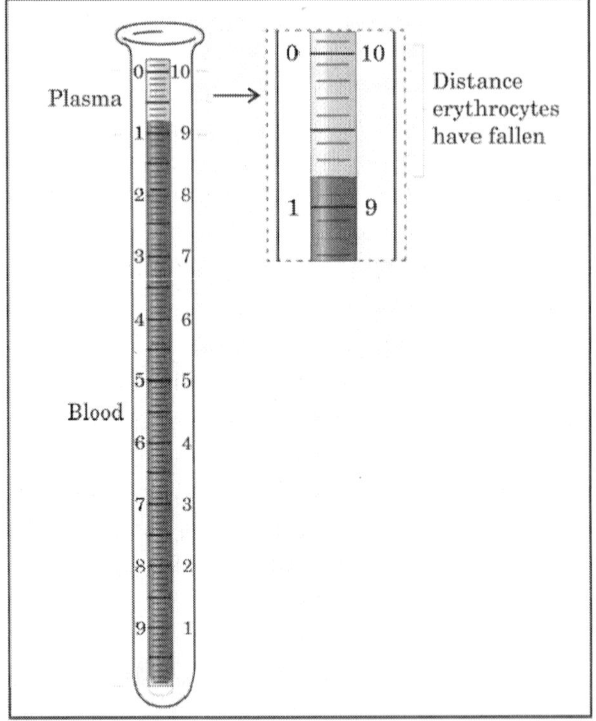

Fig. 17.1: Wintrobe's tube and its filling

- Wintrobe's tube
- Wintrobe's stand

PROCEDURE

1. Mix the blood is anti-coagulated with EDTA thoroughly.
2. By using Pasteur pipette, fill the Wintrobe's tube upto '0' mark. There should be no bubbles in the blood.
3. Place the tube vertically in ESR stand and leave undisturbed for 1 hour.
4. At the end of 1 hour, read the result.

Normal Value

For males: 0–9 mm/hr

For females: 0–20 mm/hr

Westergren's Method

It is better method than Wintrobe's method. The reading obtained is magnified as the column is lengtheir. The Westregren tube is open at both ends. It is *30 cm in length* and *2.5 mm in diameter*. The lower 20 cm are marked with 0 at the top and 200 at the buttom. It contains about 2 ml of blood.

REQUIREMENTS

- Anticoagulated blood (0.4 ml of 3.13% trisodium citrate solution + 1.6 ml blood)
- Westergren tube
- Westergren stand
- Rubber bulb (sucker)

Blood collection

Non-hemolyzed blood is anti-coagulated with EDTA at collection. It is recommended that the EDTA sample is tested within 4 hours after collection, but it has been reported that storage for up to 24 hours at 4°C still results in a stable ESR value. When ready to test, the blood sample is thoroughly mixed and diluted 4:1 using a sodium citrate solution.

Tube handling

The Westergren method uses standardized colorless, circular glass or plastic tubes, with an inner diameter of at least 2.55 mm and sufficient length to include a 200 mm sedimentation scale. The inner diameter should be constant (± 5%) over the whole length; a so called.

Westergren tube

The diluted sample is aspirated and transferred to the Westergren tube. The Westergren tube is then placed in a stable, vertical position at a constant temperature (} 1°C) between 18°C and 25°C

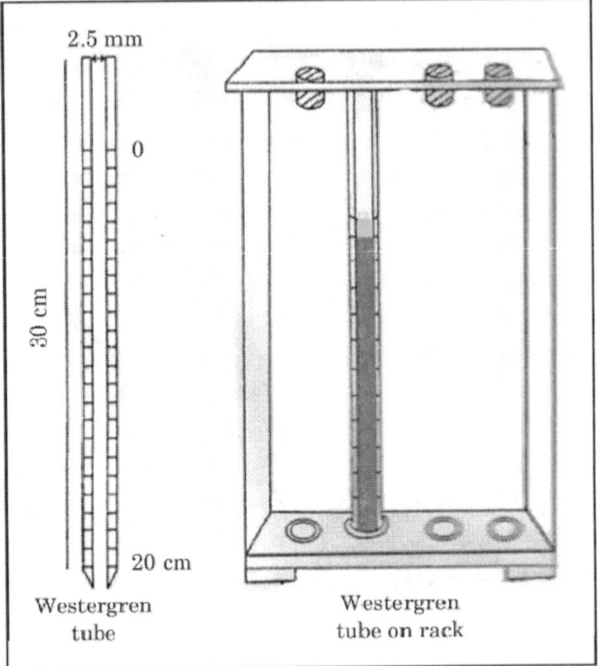

Fig. 17.2: Westregren tube and its placement

in an area free from vibrations, drafts and direct sunlight (Fig. 17.2).

Reading the result

After 60 ±1 minute, the distance from the bottom of the plasma meniscus to the top of the descended erythrocytes is read and recorded in mm. The buffy coat that is made up of leukocytes should not be included in the erythrocyte column.

Normal Value

For males: 0-10 mm/hr

For females: 0-15 mm/hr

OBSERVATIONS AND RESULTS

Note that if there is no hemolysis, there is a sharp line of demarcation between the red cells and the clear, cell-free, and straw-colored plasma. The bore of the pipette if not less than 2 mm has no effect on ESR, but inclination from the vertical gives false high values. Higher values are also obtained at extremes of temperature, in anemia, and after ingesting food.

***Sources of Error*:** These include: tilting of the tube and high temperature lead to high values while low temperature gives false low values. Hemolysed blood may obscure the sharp line separating red cells and the plasma.

Clinical Significance of ESR

The erythrocyte sedimentation rate (ESR) is a non-specific test. It is raised in a wide range of infectious, inflammatory, degenerative, and malignant conditions associated with changes in plasma proteins, particularly increases in fibrinogen, immunoglobulins, and C-reactive protein. The ESR is also affected by many other factors including anaemia, pregnancy, haemoglobinopathies, haemoconcentration and treatment with anti-inflammatory drugs.

Experiment No. 18

Aim: To Determine of Heart Rate and Pulse Rate

***Key words*:** Heartbeat, Heart rate, Stroke volume, Methods, Measuring your resting heart rate

INTRODUCTION

Heartbeat is the sound of the valves in your heart closing as they push blood from one chamber to another. *Heart rate* is the number of times the heart beats per minute *(BPM),* and the *pulse* is the beat of the heart that can be felt in any artery that lies close to the skin. The heart beats at different rates depending on whether your body is at rest or at work. When resting, the heart rate beats an average of 72 times per minute for high school students and an average of 85 BPM for middle school students. During strenuous physical activity, your heart rate or pulse increases, sometimes to twice or more its resting rate. Your *stroke volume*, the amount of blood pumped for each heartbeat, also increases. This is because the muscles that are working demand more blood to supply them with oxygen and other nutrients.

METHODS

Heart rate is measured by counting the number of times your heart beats in one minute. One way to determine your heart rate is to manually take your pulse.

The two most common locations used to take a pulse are at the *radial artery* (Fig. 18.1) in the wrist and the *carotid artery* (Fig.

18.2) in the neck. It is best to practice locating and counting your pulse when you are at rest and again during physical activity.

Measuring the Carotid Pulse

Place the tips of the index and second fingers of one hand on the side of the neck just beside the windpipe.

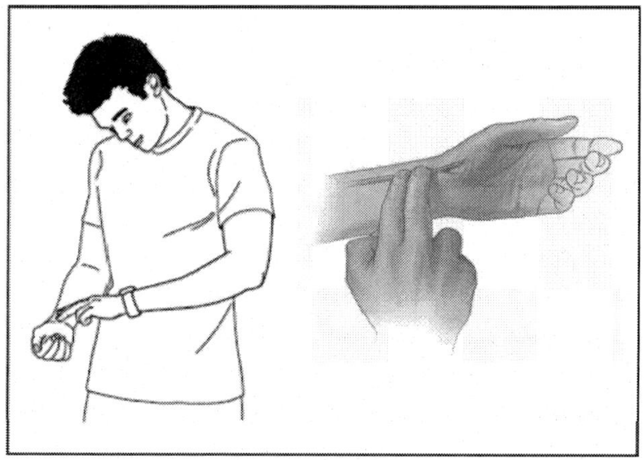

Fig. 18.1: One way to manually take pulse to measure by radial artery

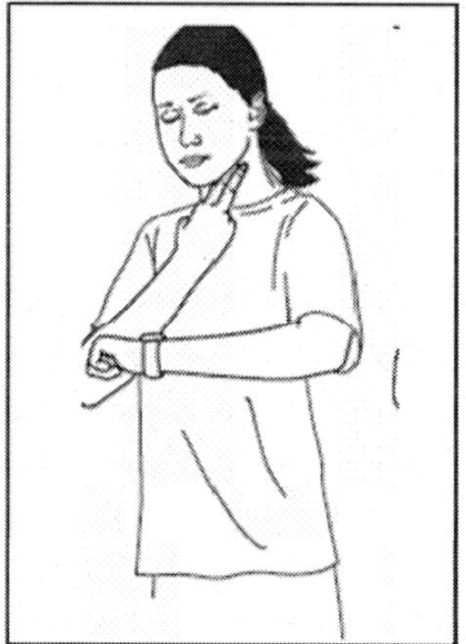

Fig. 18.2: Measuring the carotid pulse

Measuring your Resting Heart Rate

Your pulse fluctuates during the day due to activity, stress, caffeine, medications, and other actors that might influence your heart rate. A *resting pulse* is the lowest your heart rate would go during the day. You can get your best reading when you first wake up in the morning, before any activity. Relax your body, and follow the steps below for measuring your pulse.

The following are steps to take when measuring your pulse:

- ***Step One:*** Apply light to moderate pressure with the fingers until the blood pulsing beneath the fingers is felt. If no pulse is felt, move the fingers around slightly, up or down, until a pulse is felt. Do not apply excessive pressure. This may compress the artery and distort the measurement. Once the pulse is felt, move to step two.
- ***Step Two:*** Using a watch or clock with a second hand, count the number of beats felt in 30 seconds, then multiply that number by two to compute a heart rate, expressed in *BPM* (beats per minute).

Heart Rate Activity

An Example of a Resting Heart Rate

Pulse Rate (in 30 seconds): ____________ X 2 = ____________ *(beats per minute)*	Example of Resting Heart Rate: Number of beats in 30 seconds = 43 Multiply by two = 86 Resting pulse rate = 86 BPM

Take your own pulse for 30 seconds, and multiply by two.

Take your pulse six different times.

Try it three times at the carotid artery and three times at the radial artery.

Trial	*Carotid Pulse*	*Radial Pulse*
1		
2		
3		

Add all six numbers together, and divide by 6 to come up with your average.

_____ + _____ + _____ + _____ + _____ + _____ = _____ (average)
_____ divided by 6 = _____ (your average resting heart rate)

Remember this number so that you may use it later as your resting heart rate.

Resting Normal Heart Rate

Age	*Beats per minute*
Babies to age 1	100–160
Children ages 1 to 10	60–140
Children age 10+ and adults	60–100

Experiment No. 19

Aim: To Record Human Blood Pressure

***Key words*:** Blood pressure, Systolic pressure, Diastolic Pressure, Measurement principle and techniques

INTRODUCTION

Blood pressure measurement is one of the basic clinical examinations. The origin of blood pressure is the pumping action of the heart and its value depends on the relationship between cardiac output and peripheral resistance. Therefore, blood pressure is considered as one of the most important physiological variables with which to assess cardiovascular hemo-dynamics.

Blood pressure (BP) is the pressure exerted by circulating blood upon the walls of blood vessels and is one of the principal vital signs. Blood pressure is also defined, as it is the force created by the heart as it pushes blood into the arteries through the circulatory system. Each time the heart contracts or "beats" the blood is pumped out and creates a surge of pressure in the arteries. Blood pressure is the force exerted by circulating blood on the walls of blood vessels. The pressure of the circulating blood decreases as blood moves through arteries, arterioles, capillaries, and veins; the term blood pressure generally refers to *arterial pressure i.e.,* the pressure in the larger arteries, arteries being the blood vessels which take blood away from the heart. Fig. 19.1 shows the force applied to artery walls for measurement of Blood Pressure. Blood pressure usually refers to the arterial pressure of the systemic circulation, usually measured at a person's upper arm.

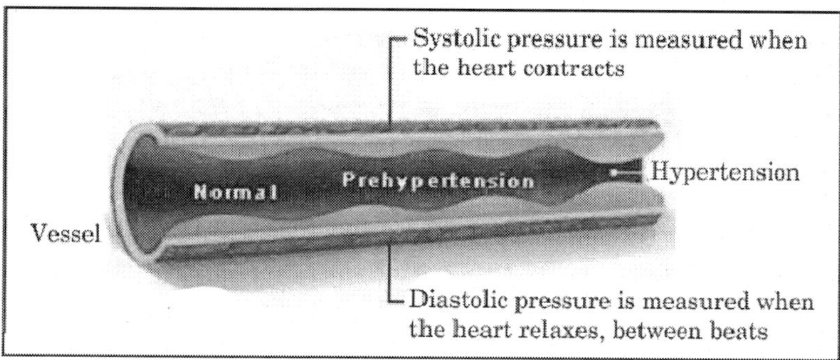

Fig. 19.1: Blood pressure and its measurement

A person's blood pressure is usually expressed in terms of the systolic pressure over diastolic pressure and is measured in millimetres of mercury. The systolic arterial pressure is defined as the peak pressure in the arteries, which occurs near the beginning of the cardiac cycle. The diastolic arterial pressure is the lowest pressure (at the resting phase of the cardiac cycle). The average pressure throughout the cardiac cycle is reported as mean arterial pressure. The pulse pressure reflects the difference between the maximum and minimum pressures measured. The blood pressure values are reported in millimetres of mercury (mmHg). (Table 19.1).

Table 19.1: Classification of blood pressure for adults

Category	*Systolic (mmHg)*	*Diastolic (mmHg)*
Hypotension	< 90	or < 60
Normal	90 – 119	and 60 – 79
Prehypertension	120 – 139	or 80 – 89
Stage 1 Hypertension	140 – 159	or 90 – 99
Stage 2 Hypertension	≥ 160	or ≥ 100

Systolic Pressure (SP)

The maximum pressure reached during peak ventricular ejection. Systolic pressure is the pressure generated when the heart contracts.

Diastolic Pressure (DP)

The minimum pressure just before beginning of ventricular ejection. Diastolic pressure is the blood pressure when the heart is relaxed.

Typical values for a resting healthy adult human are approximately 120 mmHg (16 kPa) systolic and 80 mmHg (11 kPa) diastolic written as 120/80 mmHg. These measures of arterial pressure are not static, but undergo natural variations from one heartbeat to another and throughout the day; they also change in response to stress, nutritional factors, drugs, or disease. Hypertension refers to arterial pressure being abnormally high, as opposed to hypotension, when it is abnormally low along with body temperature. The Table 19.1 shows the classification of blood pressure for adults aged 18 and older.

Pulse pressure (PP) is the difference between SP and DP, *i.e.*, PP = SP DP. The period from the end of one heart contraction to the end of the next is called the cardiac cycle. Mean pressure (MP) is the average pressure during a cardiac cycle.

Mathematically, MP can be decided by integrating the blood pressure over time. When only SP and DP are available, MP is often estimated by an empirical formula:

$$MP = DP + (PP/3) \qquad (1)$$

The values of blood pressure vary significantly during the course of 24 h according to an individual's activity. Basically, three factors, namely, the diameter of the arteries, the cardiac output, and the state or quantity of blood, are mainly responsible for the blood pressure level. When the tone increases in the muscular arterial walls so that they narrow or become less compliant, the pressure becomes higher than normal. Unfortunately, increased blood pressure does not ensure proper tissue perfusion and in some instances, such as certain types of shock, blood pressure may seem appropriate when peripheral tissue perfusion has all but stopped. The observation of blood pressures affords dynamic tracking of pathology and physiology affecting the cardiovascular system. This system in turn has profound effects on the other organs of the body.

BLOOD PRESSURE MEASUREMENT PRINCIPLE AND TECHNIQUES

Arterial pressure is most commonly measured *via* a sphygmomanometer which uses the height of a column of mercury to reflect the circulating pressure. The blood pressure is measured by means of indirect method using *sphygmomanometer* (*i.e.* sphygmo means pulse). This method is easy to use and can be automated. It can measure systolic and diastolic arterial pressure readings. Modern vascular pressure devices no longer use mercury, vascular pressure values are reported in millimetres of mercury (mmHg).

In general the Blood Pressure measurement techniques are made using two types. They are

- Direct Blood Pressure Measurement
- In- Direct Blood Pressure Measurement

Direct Blood Pressure Measurement

Direct measurement is also called Invasive measurement because bodily entry is made. Arterial blood pressure (BP) is most accurately measured invasively through an arterial line. For direct arterial blood pressure measurement an artery is cannulated or catheter. The equipment and procedure require proper setup, calibration, operation, and maintenance.

Direct blood pressure measurement is generally accepted as the gold standard of arterial pressure recording and also confers the benefit of continuous access to the artery for monitoring gas tension and blood sampling for biochemical tests. It also has the advantage of assessing cyclic variations and beat-to-beat changes of pressure continuously and permits assessment of short-term variations

Indirect Blood Pressure Measurement

Indirect measurement is often called Non-Invasive measurement because the body is not entered in the process. The upper arm, containing the brachial artery, is the most common site for indirect measurement because of its closeness to the heart and convenience of measurement, although many other sites may have been used, such as forearm or radial artery, finger, etc. Distal sites such as the wrist, although convenient to use, may give much higher systolic pressure than brachial or central sites as a result of the phenomena of impedance mismatch and reflective waves.

The most commonly used indirect methods are *Auscultation* and *Oscillometry* each is described below.

1. *Auscultator Method*

The Auscultator method most commonly employs a mercury column, an occlusive cuff and a stethoscope. The stethoscope is placed over the blood vessel for auscultation of the Korotkoff sounds, which defines both SP and DP.

First raised cuff pressure until it stopped blood circulation on the distal side of the hand, indicated by palpating the radial artery. During the following slow pressure drop, audible sounds could be heard through the stethoscope, which was placed on the skin beyond the sleeve. These sounds were affected by the blood wave in the artery under the cuff and were audible at 10-12 mmHg, slightly before the pulse could be palpated on the radial artery. At this point, cuff pressure is taken to indicate maximum blood pressure, while minimum blood pressure is achieved when the murmur sounds disappear. The appearance and disappearance of sound can be used to determine systolic and diastolic blood pressure, respectively

2. *Oscillometric Method*

In recent years, electronic pressure and pulse monitors based on oscillometry have become popular for their simplicity of use and reliability. The principle of blood pressure measurement using the oscillometric technique is dependent on the transmission of intra-arterial pulsation to the occluding cuff surrounding the limb. An approach using this technique could start with a cuff placed around the upper arm and rapidly inflated to about 30 mmHg above the systolic blood pressure, occluding blood flow in the brachial artery. The pressure in the cuff is measured by a sensor. The pressure is then gradually decreased, often in steps, such as 5 to 8 mmHg. The oscillometric signal is detected and processed at each step of pressure. The cuff pressure can also be deflated linearly in a similar fashion as the conventional auscultator method.

Equipment

For blood pressure measurements the following equipment is required

- Simple mercury sphygmomanometer,
- Stethoscope,
- Cuffs,
- Non-elastic measuring tape.

The simple mercury sphygmomanometer is recommended because there are no reliable automated devices on the market. This may change when the accuracy of future automated devices is found to be sufficient in validation against the simple mercury sphygmomanometer.

The bell of the stethoscope should be used because it gives clearer sounds than the diaphragm.

A set of 3-4 cuffs with different size should be available and special attention should be paid to the use of proper cuff width in relation to the size of the arm.

A measuring tape is used to measure arm circumference before selecting the proper cuff width.

Measurement procedures

Position of the subject

Measurements should be taken in sitting position so that the arm and back are supported. Subject's feet should be resting firmly on the floor, not dangling. If the subject's feet do not reach the floor, a platform should be used to support them.

Position of the arm

The measurements should be made on the right arm whenever possible. The subject's arm should be resting on the desk so that the antecubital fossa (a triangular cavity of the elbow joint that contains a tendon of the biceps, the median nerve, and the brachial artery) is at the level of the heart and palm is facing up. To achieve this position, either the chair should be adjusted or the arm on the desk should be raised, *e.g.* by using a pillow (Fig. 19.2). The subject must always feel comfortable.

Selection of Cuff

The greatest circumference of the upper arm is measured, with the arm relaxed and in the normal blood pressure measurement position (antecubital fossa at the level of the heart), using a non-elastic tape (Fig. 19.2). The measurement should be read to the nearest centimetre. This reading should be recorded in the data form.

Procedure

In order to carry out measurements with a sphygmometer in a reproducible way, the followings should be observed:

1. Subject should sit (or stay in the desired position) at least for 2 minutes before the measurement.
2. The inflatable cuff should be on the bare upper arm in a way that the tube runs above the brachial artery, along the crook of the arm. Upper arm should not be confined by upturned sleeves. (Fig. 19.2).

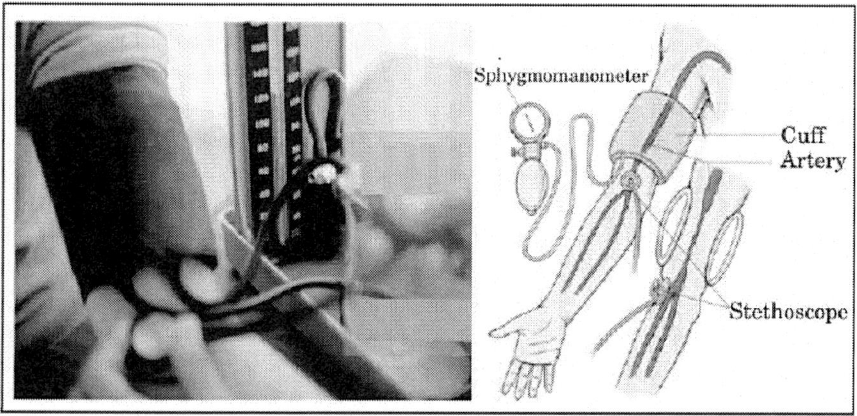

Fig. 19.2: Schematic drawing of a traditional sphygmomanometer and blood pressure measurement

3. Subject should not move or talk during the measurements.
4. Noise from the environment should be minimalised.
5. Measurements should be repeated 3 times, in a consecutive manner.

Tasks

1) Record and compare systolic and diastolic blood pressure in the left arm together with heart frequency (pulse rate) in the following body positions:
   (a) Supine (lying down)
   (b) Sitting
   (c) Standing
2) Record and analyse blood pressure and pulse rate values in a sitting position, directly following exercise (*e.g.* after 20 squats/push ups).
3) Compute and compare mean Arterial Pressure (MAP) under different experimental conditions of rest and exercise! MAP can be calculated as the value of (systolic blood pressure + 2x diastolic blood pressure)/3.

   Measured and calculated values should be recorded in the "Blood pressure" data report, along with explanations of the observed differences.

Subject Index

U

W

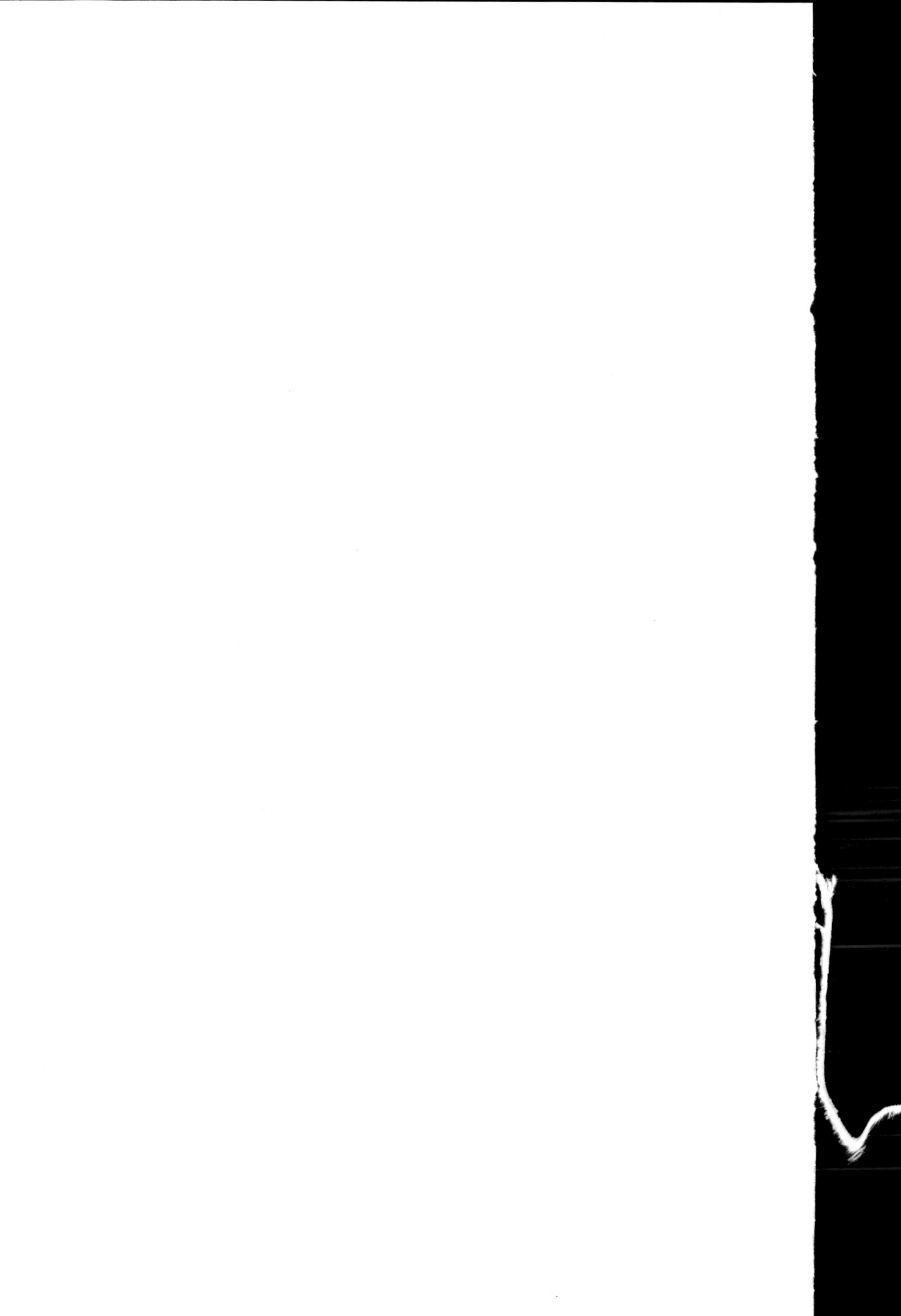